6-18-05

Sharon, Joe

may G.

and I hope this will touch
you in some way.

Craig

Tattered Flesh, Resilient Spirit

Craig H. Collison, MD

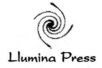

Llumina Press

Requests for permission to make copies of any part of this work should be mailed to Permissions Department, Llumina Press, PO Box 772246, Coral Springs, FL 33077-2246

ISBN: 1-59526-169-9
       1-59526-168-0
Printed in the United States of America by Llumina Press

Library of Congress Cataloging-in-Publication Data

Collison, Craig H.
Tattered flesh, resilient spirit / Craig H. Collison.
    p. cm.
    Includes bibliographical references and index.
    ISBN 1-59526-169-9 (hardcover : alk. paper) -- ISBN 1-59526-168-0 (pbk. : alk. paper)
    1. Collison, Craig H.--Health. 2. Necrotizing fasciitis--Patients--United States--Biography. 3. Pediatricians--United States--Biography. I. Title.
RC116.S84C64 2005
362.196'9298'0092--dc22   2005000579

Table of Contents

Dedication

This book is dedicated to:
the doctors who saved me,
the nurses who cared for me,
the therapists who strengthened me,
the family, friends and strangers who prayed for me,
my parents* who sacrificed so much for me,
my children who mean everything to me,
my wife who is totally devoted to me,
my God who gives life to me.

*All four of my parents

Foreword

Tattered Flesh, Resilient Spirit is a remarkable story of a young physician, Craig Collison, in the final year of his postgraduate training in Pediatrics who is suddenly faced with a life-threatening illness that strikes without warning. This biography is a straightforward and graphic account of the day-by-day struggle to survive told through the eyes of a physician, who knows all too well, the pitfalls and uncertainties of his epic battle with the "flesh-eating bacteria." What makes the book even more riveting to the reader are the personal notes, in journal form, written by his wife Michelle, family members and friends which reveal the human emotions, strength of character and depth of faith that emerge during this catastrophic series of events. Most touching are the expressions of unconditional love which are most deeply and clearly revealed during the critical and stressful times in the course of Craig's long and often painful recovery and rehabilitation. Biblical quotations are used to draw comparisons between the tenets of the Christian faith and the realities of the life experiences of this extraordinary Christian community. It will leave you, the reader, with a greater appreciation of modern medical miracles and a firmer belief in the transcendent spirit of the human person, exemplified by this remarkable young doctor and his family. You will be cheering for them as they overcome the many obstacles they face, and are healed in mind, body and spirit.

Richard B. Fratianne, MD
Professor of Surgery, Case Western Reserve University
Director Emeritus, Burn Unit, Metrohealth Medical Center, Cleveland, OH

Introduction

We as human beings are made up of two parts, flesh and spirit. We all have a physical and tangible side, skin and bones, muscle and organs. This part of us has a beginning and an end, a birth and a death. This material part of us is complemented by our spirit, our very being, the infinite part of us that can't be touched or destroyed. Our spirit is the very core of our personal existence, confined to our physical body only for our lifetime. The apostle Paul talks about the flesh and the spirit throughout his writings in the Bible. The spirit refers to both our personal spirit and to the Holy Spirit, the gift of God that works through us if we so desire.

Romans 8:10, 11 "But if Christ is in you, your body is dead because of sin, yet your spirit is alive because of righteousness. And if the Spirit of him who raised Jesus from the dead is living in you, He who raised Christ from the dead will also give life to your mortal bodies through his Spirit, who lives in you."

The contrast of flesh and spirit is a fitting theme for the story I am about to tell. As my flesh was ravaged by "flesh-eating" bacteria, any hope for survival had to come from the spirit. The flesh was failing, the odds poor, the damage great. My life was in the hands of the Spirit; the Spirit of God healing my wounds; the spirit of my wife Michelle and all the family and friends who believed in a miracle; the spirit of the doctors, nurses and therapists who refused to give up on me even when the outcome looked grim; my own spirit to fight through the pain towards recovery.

It is this incredible spirit that I wish to share with all those who read this book. I hope it especially touches those families battling similar illnesses of their own. They need to feel the power of the spirit to uplift them during their time of trial. We were supported beyond belief, buoyed up when we were sinking in despair, carried through an ordeal where so many lose the fight.

I am so fortunate, not only to be alive but to have the privilege to share our story with you. Though we are not sure how or why, a journal was started and kept at my bedside during my illness. The entries from this journal are interspersed throughout the text and take you to each moment with an intensity that would be impossible to recreate. The entries express the raw emotions of life: love, fear, death, despair, faith and hope as they happened, day-by-day. These notes are so powerful, priceless words to remember our life-changing experience. The bible verses I've inserted throughout the text are the specific verses we used to strengthen and guide us through our horrific experience.

I believe I survived my illness for many reasons, one of which was to share our story. May these words touch you in some way, strengthening your spirit, increasing your faith and hope through whatever struggle you face in your life.

Chapter 1

Background

Hebrews 4:16 Let us therefore come boldly unto the throne of grace, that we may obtain mercy, and find grace to help in time of need.

The entire saga began in April 2000. It was during the final three months of my Pediatric training program at Rainbow Babies and Children's Hospital, part of Case Western Reserve University and University Hospitals of Cleveland, in Cleveland, Ohio. This was the culmination of my training as a Pediatrician, and involved a three-year program at Rainbow after four years of medical school at The Bowman Gray School of Medicine of Wake Forest University in Winston-Salem, North Carolina. My wife Michelle was pregnant with our third child, due on my birthday, August 12th. Our boys, Taylor and Chase, were approaching their fourth and second birthdays, respectively.

Michelle and I had met and become friends at Fairbrook United Methodist Church, where both of our families attended. We got to spend a lot of time getting to know one another in youth group and youth choir. Michelle was a year older, so I never had the courage to ask her out during high school. She has always said it was a good thing that I didn't because she would have turned me down. Once we were both in college at Penn State though, I guess the age thing wasn't a big deal anymore because when I finally got up the nerve to ask, she said yes. We started dating after my freshman year and never looked back. We were engaged January 1, 1991 and got married May 31, 1992, right after my graduation from Penn State. She had graduated in December of 1991 with an Early Childhood Education degree. I had a degree in Engineering Science and Mechanics, but was headed to medical school in 1993. We both spent a year working in school settings before heading to Wake Forest. We had four great years in North Carolina with me in school and Michelle teaching kindergarten at the Salem Baptist Christian School. Our first son, Taylor, was born between my third and fourth years. After graduation, we moved to Cleveland, Ohio to continue my training in pediatrics. Michelle was able to stay home now that I had some income, and our second son, Chase, was born between my first and second years there.

After all the years of study and sleep-deprivation, everything was finally looking up. I was all set to graduate from my three-year program and move to our dream job back home in State College, Pennsylvania. Everything was ready for me to start practicing in July. We had our new home purchased in the small town of Madisonburg, in the Penns Valley region just outside of State College. The "Simon Pickel House" is a beautiful stone house which was built in 1833 and has since been completely restored. As a result of work done by the previous owners, it is on the National Register of Historic Places. We had always loved stone houses and had always hoped to own one. We were so blessed to have it happen so early in our lives. Everything that we had worked and sacrificed for was about to pay off, and the most stressful work of my residency was over. April was my last busy month. I was fortunate to have much easier rotations coming up in May and June. The movers were all lined up, our house in Cleveland had sold and spring was coming after a long winter. We weren't financially rich, but the prospect of working less, making more money and the chance to move home to central Pennsylvania after seven years of training away had us very excited. Due to the closing dates of both of our houses, Michelle, the kids, and all our stuff were to move to Pennsylvania at the end of May. I was planning to commute on weekends for a month and then move home to Pennsylvania permanently at the end of June.

Sometime during the previous summer, in 1999, I had noticed a small lump on the backside of my left shoulder, right next to my shoulder blade. I ignored it for a while, but it continued to get more noticeable. I wasn't sure what was going on; at first I began to think that my shoulder blade was just winging out at the bottom. This is caused by weakness of the muscles or nerves in that area. I had injured that shoulder significantly while playing football in college, and I assumed that the winging was a result of that. My shoulder would sometimes give me pain whenever I would stress it working, lifting weights or even just exercising. I was having trouble getting a good feel of the area since it was in such a difficult location. My schedule was crazy and the last thing that I wanted to do was go to the doctor, but Michelle finally convinced me to go. To my surprise, my doctor felt that it was probably a lipoma, a benign and common fatty tumor, but she wanted to be sure and ordered a CT scan. As she had suspected, the CT scan detected a lipoma the size of a tennis ball located under my left latissimus muscle. I was referred to Dr. Goldstein, one of the plastic surgeons at the hospital where I was training. He agreed with the diagnosis and was willing to surgically remove the lipoma. Because it was located under muscle, the surgery would require general anesthesia, but could be done in one to two hours, allowing me to go home the same day. I really wanted to have the procedure done during the winter so it wouldn't hamper my chances of golfing in the spring. As is often the case, my insurance company initially denied paying for the procedure, claiming that it was only cosmetic. After a second letter describing my discomfort, they agreed to cover the procedure. All this took time though. The soonest we could schedule the surgery was April 20, which was the day after and two days before being "on-call" as a supervising resident at Rainbow. Two days wasn't a lot of time for recovery, but I really wanted to recuperate enough to golf with all my friends and colleagues before we all went our separate ways in July.

Everything went as planned on the day of my surgery. Our friends were able to watch Taylor and Chase so that Michelle could spend the day at the hospital with me. The lipoma was removed without any difficulty. A drain was left in the wound to alleviate the collection of fluid or blood at the surgery site. The operation was deemed a success, and Michelle and I went home later that afternoon with some pain medicine and the knowledge that I was going to be uncomfortable for a while. Michelle was to empty the drain bulb on a regular basis and keep track of its volume. Dr. Goldstein was able to remove the lipoma without permanently destroying my latissimus muscle, the large muscle that forms the back part of your armpit, but it had taken quite a bit of work freeing the mass from the muscle. A lot of soreness was to be expected, but I was able to sleep without too much difficulty.

The next day was Good Friday. I actually felt worse than I had the night before. Sometime mid-morning I spiked my first temperature, about 102 degrees Fahrenheit. I didn't feel like eating or drinking very much, and felt pretty nauseated. I blamed this on the pain medication. I had lots of nausea but preferred mild pain to taking codeine as I had done when I had my appendix out in the spring of 1991. Michelle was quite concerned about my fever and called Dr. Goldstein. He was in clinic Friday afternoon, so he decided to have me come in so he could look at my wound. The car ride was real torture on my shoulder, and I was feeling pretty weak so Michelle got me into a wheelchair for the long walk from the parking garage to the clinic. I wasn't worried at this point as I expected to be sore, and I knew that it was relatively common to have some fever after any surgery. Dr. Goldstein agreed with me and felt the wound looked fine, so we went home. Michelle's parents arrived Friday night to celebrate Easter with us. I wasn't very good company, and stayed on the couch all evening. I started vomiting off and on that evening, and had an episode of the shakes. I couldn't stop shivering. I still thought this was from the Percocet, the pain medicine I was taking. As much as I didn't want to, I finally conceded that I wasn't going to able to take my call at the hospital on Saturday, so I called the chief resident to let her know that a replacement would have to be found. There were always backups that were on "Jeopardy" call to fill in for sick residents. This occurred during a resident's easier months, when they didn't have any other call responsibilities. I really hated having to dump my shift on one of my colleagues, but it was becoming increasingly obvious that I wouldn't have the strength to work. That night was extremely difficult. My fever kept going higher and higher. By this time, Michelle was beside herself with worry. I kept reassuring her that I would be fine and I just needed a little time until I started feeling better.

Matthew 17:20 (Jesus speaking) "Because you have so little faith. I tell you the truth, if you have faith as small as a mustard seed, you can say to this mountain, 'Move from here to there' and it will move. Nothing will be impossible for you."

Chapter 2

Emergency Room

S aturday brought me more of the same misery, no relief as I had hoped. We expected the fever to start to subside, but it continued to soar as high as 105 degrees F. I still didn't think that this was anything out of the ordinary. Michelle, however, was of the opposite mind-set. She had a sense that this was developing into a major problem. I could tell that she was growing increasingly concerned. I did my best to remain calm, and tried to cope with feeling so miserable. I'm sure it was a combination of my eternal optimism, pain medications and high fever, but I wasn't panicking. This is one reason why doctors should not be their own physician whenever possible. It is difficult to make critical decisions about your own care even when you are healthy.

I was used to being around catastrophe, taking care of sick kids in a large referral hospital. I saw bad things happening to children and their families all the time. I had seen kids who had gone to sleep feeling fine and never woke up. I had seen kids devastated and dying from cancer and leukemia. I had seen kids hurt, killed in car accidents, or burned in fires. Even with all my experience of the worst that life has to offer, I never once believed that I would be the victim of an equally devastating illness.

My head remained optimistic, but my body was in shambles.

I was getting so weak that I had trouble supporting my own weight. Walking ten feet to the bathroom exhausted me. I was still vomiting and having trouble keeping anything down, so it was hard to push myself to drink knowing it would come right back up. The fluid that was coming from the drain in my wound continued and even seemed to pick up a little. It really didn't change in consistency or color, remaining a thin red fluid. Respecting my doctor's family time, I didn't want to call him again, but I finally relented and let Michelle call early Saturday afternoon. I had vomited some bile, black-green nasty vomit that indicated my bowel had stopped moving things through. The bile is made by the liver, stored in the gall bladder, and is evident in vomit only when it backs up into the stomach from a lack of action. Seeing bile is never a good thing and it scared both of us enough to prompt her to call. After Michelle and Dr. Goldstein discussed the situation, he decided that I should come into the Emergency Room for some IV fluids, a wound check and possible admission to the hospital. Dr. Namuri, the plastic surgery fellow who assisted in my original surgery, would see me in the ER and decide what I needed. Dr. Goldstein was mostly concerned at that time that I was becoming dehydrated from all of the vomiting.

I had mixed feelings about going to the ER. I knew some IV fluids would help me feel better, but I also knew how tortuous the ride to the hospital would be. Michelle had to help me get some semblance of clothing on. Michelle's father had to help me down one and a half flights of stairs to get to the car. I was weak and lightheaded and had intense pain in my shoulder. I couldn't get comfortable sitting, but I had no other choice short of calling an ambulance. It was the longest four-mile ride of my life. Every bump along the way brought tears to my eyes from the ever-worsening pain.

I Peter 5:7 "Cast all your care upon Him; for He careth for you."

Upon our arrival at the University Hospitals ER, one of the security guards was nice enough to get a wheelchair for me and wheeled me inside while Michelle parked the car. I started filling out the registration paperwork but was so relieved when Michelle arrived to take over. Once I was registered, I was taken to the triage area so a nurse could check my vital signs. She found I had a fever of about 103 degrees, low blood pressure at 90/60, and tachycardia with my heart rate 120-130 (normal 60-80). The nurse had a difficult time getting my blood pressure, it took her several attempts before she got a reading. I was hoping that I looked sick enough that they would take me right to a bed, but unfortunately we were sent back to the waiting room. I was not happy, looking awful, feeling awful, and trying not to vomit. We were surrounded by sick people in the very same ER where I worked. I was hoping not to be recognized. I'm not sure how long it took to get me into an ER bed, but it felt like an eternity. What a relief it was to lie down in that bed. I could finally rest and didn't have to sit up.

Once I was taken back to a bed, my nurse quickly got me settled, drew some blood and put in an IV to get some much needed fluid into me. They obtained a complete blood count, also known as a CBC, electrolytes, and a blood culture. In what seems remarkable to me in retrospect, this CBC was normal, without any evidence of my body mobilizing to fight an infection. This original blood culture from the ER never grew any bacteria, subsequent ones would grow Group A Strep. I had been feverish for over 24 hours at that point, so it seems that my blood-work should have been more conclusive regarding what was going on. My vital signs demonstrated that an infection was raging inside of me, causing my high fever, vomiting and low blood pressure. In contrast, the blood count gave the impression that I was likely suffering from a stomach virus. If my white blood cells, those cells that fought infection, had been elevated at this point, giving the doctors clear evidence that I needed immediate surgical intervention, would things have been done differently? Could my personal devastation have been avoided or reduced? My particular situation and others I have seen as a physician reiterate the fact that the patient's condition must be valued first and foremost. Laboratory findings and imaging are tools to assist physicians in the diagnosis, but don't always give clear or timely information.

Not long after I got settled, Dr. Namuri came by and looked at my wound. He still thought it looked fine, but thought I should be admitted for hydration. After seeing me and my lab work, he spoke to Dr. Goldstein who agreed with the plan. After a couple of hours in the ER, we were admitted to a post-operative floor for more fluids and rest.

Proverbs 3:3, 5-8 "Let love and faithfulness never leave you; bind them around your neck, write them on the tablet of your heart. Trust in the Lord with all your heart and lean not on your own understanding; in all ways acknowledge him, and he will make your paths straight. Do not be wise in your own eyes; fear the Lord and shun evil. This will bring health to your body and nourishment to your bones."

Chapter 3

Flesh Eating Bacteria

Once I was moved from the ER to the post-operative floor, Michelle and I waited hours for the resident doctor to come and officially admit me. The resident for plastic surgery was also covering for cardio-thoracic surgery patients that night, and as they were having difficulty with a patient on that service, we waited. I didn't feel well but was content to lie still in my bed and rest. At approximately 11:00 PM, I convinced Michelle that she should go home and get some sleep. I felt bad that she had spent all this time with me, especially with her parents at home with the kids. She was concerned with my lower blood pressure and continued fever, but she reluctantly gave in and went home. While it was hard for me to believe I could get any worse, after she left, I did. The pain in my back had gotten to the point that I couldn't stand it any more. I just could not get comfortable and continuously rolled from side to side without any relief. The pain got to be too much and I called the nurse in. I told her that she needed to get somebody to see me quickly. I had been ignoring all the signs, but was finally convinced that something was very wrong. At that point even with all the IV fluid I had been given, my blood pressure had dropped so low that the nurse could only get 60/palp, undetectable or zero, with multiple attempts. This is where my memory becomes a blur. My story for the subsequent three weeks is what I have pieced together from Michelle's notes, doctor's notes and other people's memories. I suspect that the reason I can't remember further details from that night was that I was given pain medicine to relieve my unbearable pain, and this had knocked me out.

Around 4:15 in the morning, Easter Sunday, five hours after leaving me, Michelle received a phone call from Dr. Goldstein. He had been called in to check on me as the result of my worsening condition. He told Michelle he was taking me to the operating room to open things back up. He suspected a wound infection was the cause for my pain, fever and deteriorating clinical state. On the phone he asked her how fast she could get there and if she wanted to talk to me before they took me to the operating room. She said it would take her twenty minutes and that she did want to talk to me. He told her they couldn't wait that long and needed to get me prepped for surgery. He would get her in to see me in the pre-op area if she could get there in time.

I can only speculate about Dr. Goldstein's thoughts as he took me to surgery early Easter morning. What he found when he opened me back up was the worst case of all the possibilities, the most feared of wound infections. He found inflammation, pus, and most concerning of all, the evidence of necrosis in the area where my lipoma had been removed. As a result of their findings, the diagnosis of necrotizing fasciitis and myositis was made. This diagnosis was truly dreadful, as a summary of published medical reports puts the mortality rate from necrotizing fasciitis with muscle involvement, myositis, at 80-100%.[1] This means that in some of these patient-groups studied there were no survivors at all. At best, the hope for survival for any patient with this diagnosis was only 20%.

Necrotizing fasciitis and myositis is an infection of the fascia, soft tissue, and muscle by a bacteria called *Streptococcus pyogenes*, more commonly known as strep. There are several groups within this species, and they are labeled A through G. Different groups have different characteristics and cause different diseases. For example, Group B Strep is a bacteria found normally in 40% of women's birth canals, and only causes potential problems for infants born through an infected canal. Group A Strep includes the bacteria which cause strep throat, scarlet fever, rheumatic fever and also necrotizing fasciitis and myositis. There are a few other bacteria which can also cause the necrotizing infection, but Group A Strep is by far the most common. Known through the press as the "flesh-eating" bacteria, the strep in those cases is extremely aggressive and often deadly for its victim. As it infects soft tissues, it kills healthy human cells at an incredible speed, leaving dead cells in its wake. This tissue turns a black color, which is then referred to as necrotic tissue. The name necrotizing fasciitis and myositis means that the infection causes inflammation of the fascia and muscle, rapidly killing its cells leaving dead, necrotic tissue.

Why is this particular bacteria so much more aggressive and deadly than other bacteria that cause wound infections? There are several factors which add to its lethal nature to our cells. First, it releases many toxins that are extremely damaging to cells it comes into contact with, causing rapid destruction. These toxins are also delivered to the rest of the body through the bloodstream, causing decreases in blood pressure and can eventually send the victim into shock. Secondly, the flesh-eating bacteria have a defense mechanism to defeat neutrophils, white blood cells that fight infection, sent by the host's immune system to the site of infection.

Neutrophils are our body's main defense against bacteria. Antibodies, which come from lymphocytes, another type of white blood cell, are geared more towards fighting viruses and fungi, while the neutrophils are the best defense against bacteria.

In a bacterial infection, a signal from the site of infection triggers a release of neutrophils from the bone marrow and from resting places on the walls of blood vessels. This process, called demargination, is where these neutrophils that are hanging onto vessel walls get the signal to release and follow the signal to the site of the invading bacteria. As more of these neutrophils are in the bloodstream, they can be detected on a complete blood count. The patterns seen in neutrophils and all the different types of white blood cells can give a good indication that an infection is occurring. Based on the distribution of the different types of white blood cells, determination of what type of infection, ie. bacterial versus viral can sometimes be seen. My white blood-cell count taken in the emergency room didn't show an increase in neutrophils indicative of a serious bacterial infection. Unfortunately, this was misleading to those taking care of me.

When these neutrophils arrive at the infection site, their job is to engulf bacteria, then kill them. The Group A Strep is able to thwart this response in a mechanism that isn't totally understood. In recent research, scientists have shown that the strep can stimulate up to 400 more genes than other bacteria within the neutrophil, causing it to self-destruct before it can do its job. Without the neutrophil defense-mechanism, the strep is able to multiply rapidly and spread through tissues at an incredible pace.

As Dr. Goldstein opened up my wounds and learned the horrible truth, there was no time to lose. The only effective treatment for necrotizing fasciitis and myositis is surgical removal of the infected and necrotic tissue. The tissue removal needs to get ahead of the bacteria in order to stop the progression of destruction. For the next 20 hours, Dr. Goldstein and other surgeons did just that, desperately trying to get ahead of the infection while I still had enough tissue to survive. Antibiotics by themselves are ineffective in treating necrotizing fasciitis, but are used as an adjunct to the crucial debridement. The affected tissues must be surgically cut away for there to be any hope of surviving the "flesh-eating" bacteria.

With my survival hanging in the balance, the surgeons started removing tissue near my posterior left axilla. They kept dissecting through layers of skin, nerves, blood vessels, fat and even muscle. As they described it, the infection progressed so fast that they could see the advancement "right before their eyes." Similar to removing a tumor, the goal of the surgery was to cut away all the affected tissue until normal, healthy tissue was reached on all the borders. Obviously, everything that was healthy and could be saved was beneficial to me long-term, but they had to get the dead infected tissue completely removed or I was a goner. The surgeons followed the progression of the infection down my left side from the left armpit, in some areas from my sternum all the way around to my spine. As the disease spread down my left flank, the surgeons found the deadly bacteria burrowing across my stomach below the belly button. This is when Dr. Goldstein called in an abdominal specialist, Dr. Shenk, to help as they didn't know how far or how deep the infection would invade. Dr. Shenk was a great help, keeping them working fast as the infection continued around to a large patch on my right flank. For brief breaks, the surgeons would leave the operating room to update Michelle and the rest of my family and to take a quick breather. They couldn't leave the operating room for long though, they had to keep working as the "flesh-eating" bacteria continued to advance.

Isaiah 41:10 "Fear thou not; for I am with thee: be not dismayed; for I am thy God: I will strengthen thee; yea, I will help thee."

As the day went on, the despair and severity of my catastrophic illness really hit home for those around me. My parents arrived from Mississippi mid-afternoon on Easter, still unsure of how or what was really going on. Residents and faculty from Rainbow were notified of the situation and began arriving to provide any support they could. As the surgery stretched into the evening hours Easter Sunday night, word came from the operating room. While the infection had been previously only traveling down away from my armpit, the surgeons suddenly found that it was spreading upwards into my neck. This was such devastating news, with the frightening thought of my neck and possibly my head and face being eaten alive. Would my face be totally disfigured as the bacteria showed me no mercy?

With no choice but to keep going, the surgeons called for an ear, nose and throat doctor to help with the neck dissection. The stakes were so high as they worked feverishly to save my head and neck. Despair mounted when news of the spread into my neck came into the ICU waiting room. Those present spontaneously gathered together in a circle. Through the tears and fear of what was to come, everyone prayed, fervently asking for a miracle. Michelle describes the incredible power and strength everyone took away from that circle. Unable to do anything to directly save me, they all lifted me up. They called on the Spirit, the God of mercy to save me. Not long after this circle time, word again came from the operating room that the progression had been stopped and my face and head had been spared. The doctors had cut away a great deal of soft tissue, but all the crucial components of my neck had been saved. The prayers from that circle of family and friends were directly answered, the Spirit was alive and working hard on my behalf. I still had a fighting chance and would live to see another day.

James 5:14-15 "Is any one of you sick? He should call the elders of the church to pray over him and anoint him with oil in the name of the Lord. And the prayer offered in faith will make the sick person well; the Lord will raise him up. If he has sinned, he will be forgiven. Therefore confess your sins to each other and pray for each other so that you may be healed. The prayer of a righteous man is powerful and effective."

After a staggering amount of surgery to remove the infected tissue, the team felt confident that the progression had finally been stopped. I had survived 20 hours of surgery, anesthesia, blood loss and infection. Everyone was physically and emotionally drained, but relieved in a sense that I had lived through such an ordeal. The first battle of what was to be a long war had been won. The losses were great. My flesh, ravaged by infection and surgery, was a mere semblance of what it was. But making it through to this point was such a miracle that these defects seemed almost insignificant, a small price to pay for my life.

Chapter 4

Intensive Care Unit

After the grueling surgery that had consumed the majority of the previous 24 hours, I was taken back to the ICU, heavily bandaged, intubated and still on the ventilator. This happened about five o'clock a.m. on Monday morning. Dr. Goldstein and all the members of the surgical team were exhausted but encouraged that they finally appeared to have gotten ahead of the bacteria. Despite their successes, they also knew that even if they had cleared my body of the "flesh-eating" bacteria, the surgery was only the beginning.

Michelle and some other friends and family were able to come in and see me shortly after I was settled back in my room in the intensive care unit. Remarkably, after all the surgery and anesthesia I had been through, I was able to partially wake up and communicate with Michelle. I couldn't talk since I had a breathing tube protruding through my vocal cords, so I resorted to using my finger and drawing letters on the palm of her hand to spell words to her. Looking back, I can vaguely recall doing some of this, but I'm not able to place at what point during the ordeal it happened. From notes in Michelle's journal, she wrote that I was concerned about her and the kids. After having a portable x-ray taken, I was very concerned that she had left during the x-ray to avoid exposing our unborn baby to any radiation. At one point, I also spelled out P L U G. Michelle and my dad finally figured out after some frustration, that I was telling them that I had a mucous plug in either my breathing tube or lungs that needed to be suctioned. I do remember being very frustrated trying to adopt this new form of communication. Feeling as poorly as I did, I couldn't hide my temper.

By Michelle's report, my body was incredibly swollen from all the fluids and blood products that had been given to me throughout my lengthy surgery. While normally a good size man, I was enormous, swelled almost beyond recognition. I was so big that my shoulders were touching both sides of my full size hospital bed, my hands and feet had more than doubled in size. Slits were all that were visible of my eyes. In addition to my altered body state, I was hooked up to a noisy ventilator, multiple IV and central lines, and seemingly countless monitors which constantly flashed and beeped. By all accounts the entire scene was not pretty, even disturbing to many of my visitors. My swelling had gotten so bad that fluid literally oozed out of my skin so briskly that a steady drip was rolling off of my bed and hitting the floor. The doctors were fighting a losing battle with my fluid status. I was losing so much fluid through my gaping wounds and even intact skin. All they could do was to constantly give me more fluid intravenously, keeping enough blood pumping to my vital organs. This vicious cycle continued, and wouldn't end until my wounds and blood vessels healed enough to slow down their leaking.

Through my multiple IV access sites, I was continuing on IV fluids, blood products, and several medications. One of the several medicines was known as a pressor, which acted to keep my blood pressure up high enough to allow blood to perfuse my organs. The bacteria in my blood stream were releasing toxins that caused my vessels to dilate, decreasing blood pressure. These pressor medicines were given to counteract that dilation. These medications are used frequently for the very ill in any ICU to aid the heart and the blood vessels in functioning even while they are at sub-optimal strength. I was also on several high-powered antibiotics to help fight residual infection in my blood and anywhere else it might be hiding. Even though all Group A Strep, including the "flesh-eating" bacteria, are uniformly sensitive to penicillin, in life or death situations, such as I was in, the doctors weren't taking any chances.

At a family meeting late Monday, Dr. Goldstein discussed the successes they had in the operating room, and also talked about the difficult times that were ahead. Their biggest worries were that my lungs would fill with fluid as the rest of my body had, and that my kidneys would fail, due to the overload of proteins from my massive tissue destruction. My family was left with the statement that the next 24 hours would be critical to my survival. Dr. Goldstein also recommended that my brothers hastily make their way to see me, emphasizing the urgency and my low likelihood of surviving the next assault on my body. Short of hearing that your loved one has died, these are probably the most difficult words to hear from your doctor. During the first week after my major surgery, the doctors at University Hospitals had to say "if we can get through the next 24 hours" more than once, frustrating everyone, especially my mom. As I survived through the said 24 hours, my family expected that to mean I was supposed to be better and out of critical danger. Unfortunately, the nature of my illness continuously bombarded me with deadly threats.

Survival in the ICU is dependent on many factors. Generally speaking, patients with one specific-ailment that affects only one organ-system have a much greater chance of survival. Unfortunately, as most disease processes progress, more and more organ systems become involved, increasing the severity of illness and the difficulties of treatment. As a result, the likelihood of survival decreases with every additional organ-system that is involved and failing. This was what happened in my case. It began as just an infection, but progressed to include respiratory failure, circulatory system failure, kidney failure, and endocrine failure. Once three or more systems begin to fail, the chance of survival falls to under 20 percent. Not only did I have less than a one in five chance of surviving the necrotizing fasciitis and myositis, I was now heading towards a second set of the same poor odds based on my multiple organ failures.

John 3:16 "For God so loved the world that he gave his only begotten Son, that whoever believes in Him shall not perish but have everlasting life."

As the doctors had expected, my overall condition worsened over the next few days. My lungs were filling with fluid and I was developing a condition known as ARDS, Adult Respiratory Distress Syndrome. As the blood vessels in my lungs became weaker from the toxins released by the bacteria, more and more fluid was making its way into my alveoli, also known as air sacs. Because of this it was getting more difficult to adequately ventilate and oxygenate me. The fluid in the alveoli acted as a physical barrier, disrupting the diffusion of oxygen into, and carbon dioxide out of my bloodstream. To get around this barrier, the ventilator had to work harder, forcing the oxygenated air faster, more times per minute, and with higher pressure past the fluid. Frequent blood-gas measurements were taken to show the doctors how my body was responding to the ventilator Adjustments were then made with the ventilator based on those results. A blood gas tells you the pH, acid or base, pCO2 and pO2, the positive pressure of each gas within the blood, bicarbonate and oxygen saturation. These all interact in a complex manner to give a good picture of how the ventilator is working.

Michelle received a crash course in ventilator management from my resident friends and began to understand the basics of what was going on. Although she had no medical background, she quickly learned about good and bad blood-gas values, along with lab results and vital signs. This made her feel like she knew how I was truly doing. Later in my illness, after our transfer to Metrohealth Hospital, the nurses there were amazed at how well she understood all the different values and were surprised to learn that other than during my illness, she had not received any medically training. This was one of Michelle's coping mechanisms, constantly getting my numbers gave her a positive "job" to do in the midst of all the tears and worry.

My kidney function was also in a steady decline. The kidney, explained in basic terms, is a blood filter, working to excrete waste, maintain normal electrolyte levels, and manage blood pressure. Just as any filter that gets plugged by larger particles, the breakdown components of my muscle and skin, destroyed by the flesh-eating bacteria, did just that. This plugging effect coupled with the decreased blood flow to my kidneys from all the fluid losses led to a steady decrease in my glomerular filtration rate, GFR. When the blood isn't being filtered fast enough, this causes problems for the entire body. This can potentially include waste buildup, electrolyte abnormalities and blood-pressure problems. There is a lab test that measures a compound known as creatinine. This test is a way for physicians to follow kidney function. As my condition worsened, my creatinine went from the normal range, 0.8-1.2, up to 3.1. Creatinine is a compound from muscle, filtered by the kidneys at a known rate and therefore gives a comparative picture of how the kidney filtering is working. The jump in value from the normal range to 3.1 may not seem too bad at first glance, except that creatinine is a logarithmic lab value, meaning that every increase of 1 is an increase by a factor of 10. For example, if you're creatinine goes from 1 to 2, it doesn't double but rather goes up by a factor of 10, which means the kidney function is 10 times worse than normal at a creatinine of 2. In my case, this meant that at a creatinine of 3.1, my kidneys were working at worse than 1/100th of their usual capabilities. A creatinine of 4 would correspond to filtering decreased to 1/1000th of normal. This is a very serious impairment, and talk from the medical team was beginning to move toward using dialysis to assist my kidney function.

My gaping wounds were another problem confronting the ICU team. The care of these wounds was a very difficult and time-consuming task for the surgeons and nurses. University Hospitals lacks the facilities of a burn unit equipped with spray tables to easily clean and dress large wounds, so this procedure had to be done in my hospital bed. It took up to three hours for each dressing-change, and this was being done every eight hours round-the-clock. By this time I was mostly comatose and unable to assist the staff, so I had to be lifted and moved to get to all of my wound sites. With all the extra fluid on board, my weight was in the neighborhood of 250 pounds, which made things even more difficult for them. This was in addition to my breathing tube and multiple IV and central lines that had to be kept in place while I was moved. What a difficult task it was for the staff.

Skin is such an essential part of each person's health, it is taken for granted until you lose it. Skin serves many functions for us, as a barrier to infection, and a regulator of body temperature and fluid status. As I described before, my bed in the intensive care unit was continually dripping onto the floor from all the fluid that leaked out of my wounds. A common problem with such large wounds is yeast infections, so I was started on some antifungal medications once that became a problem. Yeast loves moist areas with decreased oxygen-content, my covered wounds combined with the multiple antibiotics I was on contributed to a bad infection. The yeast infections continued to be a menace that would be dealt with off and on throughout my entire illness.

The other organ-system receiving medical attention was my endocrine system. Our endocrine system is the mechanism that deals with all the hormones and metabolism that occurs in our bodies. In response to distress, our bodies secrete increased amounts of different steroids from the adrenal glands to help the body and its cells with all of its defense mechanisms. One of the side effects of this increased steroid production is increased blood sugars. This was another of my lab values the ICU team was watching closely. At the most critical time, they were checking my blood sugar every hour. As my blood sugars continued to increase due to this steroid effect, I was even given some injectable insulin to control my blood sugar, just a diabetic would do.

Juggling all of these different ailments at the same time was very challenging and required continual assistance and decision making by the ICU physicians. They had to worry about each organ system both individually and as they interacted together. They had to make sure that an intervention in one organ system wouldn't worsen the function of another. As a patient with such a devastating illness, I was fortunate to be part of the 20 percent who survive multiple-organ shutdown. Once the infection was stopped, the ICU staff was able to keep me alive and support my organ systems that were failing, long enough for them to recover. Why did I survive when others don't? Was it the fact that I was young? Was it the fact that I had great doctors? Was it the fact that I didn't smoke? Was it that I had more people praying for me or that they were praying harder? Was it the fact that I had a stronger will to survive? Was it luck? To this day I still grapple with these questions, knowing full-well all of these issues played some role in my recovery.

Psalm 33:20-22 "We wait in hope for the Lord; He is our help and our shield. In Him our hearts rejoice, for we trust in his holy name.

May your unfailing love rest upon us, O Lord; even as we put our hope in you."

By early evening on Monday, a large number of people had arrived in town to see and support us. All four of our parents were there. Also present were my brothers Keith and Eric, as well as Michelle's sister Heather and her husband Donnie. Our friends from North Carolina, Paul and Laurel, had arrived late Sunday night, and our friends from Cleveland, Dan and Rhonda, had come back early from an Easter trip to Michigan to be with us. Later that week John and Amy flew in from South Carolina to support us, and Russ and Linda came over from Pennsylvania. On top of all this support, the residents and faculty from Rainbow were there at the ICU round-the-clock, checking on me, bringing meals, picking up people at the airport, etc. This was in addition to their already exhausting work schedules. With John and Leron in charge, they were there doing everything they could to help, continually assisting Michelle and the rest of my family in keeping tabs on my condition. With my lab values available on the hospital computer, all of my colleagues were following along with them, even to the point where they were seeing them faster than the ICU team. It had gotten to the point that the ICU team had asked Dr. Avner, our pediatric department chair, to have everyone back off a bit as they were getting too involved. How great to be so cared for.

As a result of all my supporters, the ICU waiting room was basically taken over by my friends and family. Twenty-four hours a day, the vigil was present, with many people staying with Michelle overnight. The average was about ten people there for me at any one time. The nurses and staff in the ICU were great to them, even providing pillows and blankets to anyone who needed them. The phone in the ICU waiting room seemed to constantly ring, usually someone looking for an update on my condition or relaying a message. This overwhelming presence gave our group a unique experience; to meet, share and even pray with other ICU patient's family and friends, and with countless hospital staff. We hope that the strong show of support from our group served as a positive example of our faith and love to all those around us.

What a test of faith it was, within a few days our lives had fallen from a wonderful high to this horrible battle with death. We were at the end of a residency, ready to move on to a new job in a new house and ready to have our third baby. Now, I was suddenly overcome with an infection from "flesh-eating" bacteria, leaving me terribly wounded and with little hope of survival. Fortunately, I was in a world-class medical facility with the best team of physicians and staff doing everything they could. What else could be done? My family and friends prayed. Prayer was the one thing that my friends and family could do to help me and the doctors, and they prayed every chance they could. The prayers didn't just stay there with our group either. As word spread about our situation, hundreds and eventually thousands of people were praying for us. The prayer chain grew longer as entire churches, whose members didn't even know us personally, took our needs up to God. Our news also spread by e-mail as my friends and former classmates from State College High School and Penn State University sent out almost daily updates to large networks of associated people. While I wasn't awake to see it, the strength of my family and friends to put me in the hands of God the way they did must have played a part in my miraculous recovery.

Journal Entries 4/26/00

Praise God! We have hopeful news this morning from all three surgeons - Dr. Goldstein, Dr. Shenk and Dr. Stepnek. Dr. Goldstein's words are that you actually look better today - such wonderful news!!!!

"Fear thou not, for I am with thee; be not dismayed, for I am thy God: I will strengthen thee; yea, I will help thee." Isaiah 41:10

M-

Michelle and Craig:

What strength you have. Strength in your faith, strength in your relationship with each other and with family, friends and colleagues. Your ways have touched those around you and now I'm amazed to see others giving back in the most wonderful and supportive ways. Calls, visits and prayers keep coming. Each visit from a doctor on your case gives us glimmers of hope. We know you are in no way "out of the woods" but we will be patient. You must be as well. All things happen in God's time, not ours. We will put our trust in him. Each day is a blessing. Look for the brightness of sunshine, the sweet smell of spring flowers and the tenderness of love in our hearts for you. You are so precious to us. We all have so much to look forward to as a family, a new baby, a new home and a new job. Much to encourage us. We will be there to help in any way you need...please ask. Together we will look ahead to a beautiful future.

Love you bushels - Mom! (F)

Dear Craig, Michelle, Taylor, Chase and ?:

How deep is my love for you? There is truly no way to measure it or put it in words! I feel that God has shown us such love by answering all the prayers that went up for you during the critical early hours of this illness. Praise Him. I'm so proud and blessed to see such an out-pouring of love, help, and comfort from all of your friends and family. The doctors, residents and nursing staff have been so dedicated and concerned about doing the best for you and everyone is doing their best to help in your recovery. So many folks have called to offer prayers and show their concern.

I know you are strong and will do your best. You are a wonderful family with a wonderful future! "Trust in the Lord with all of your heart and lean not unto thine own understanding. In all ways acknowledge Him and He shall direct your paths." Proverbs 3:5

Love- Mom C

As the week went on, it was marked with constant ups and downs in my condition. I continued to be swollen and almost unrecognizable as my beard and mustache grew and my hair became progressively more unkept. Even though many of my organs were failing, none were broken beyond repair. The ICU team was able to keep them functioning through their interventions. I was kept asleep with pain medications, preventing me from struggling against the ventilator and blocking any pain from my open wounds. I can recall waking up at two different times during my stay in the ICU at University Hospitals. Once was while they were putting a Swan-Ganz catheter into my neck so the doctors could more accurately measure the blood pressures inside my heart and lungs. That hurt. I would have preferred to stay asleep during that procedure. Another time was while they were changing my dressings. Though I wasn't thinking clearly, I definitely remember both occurrences, especially the dressing change. One of the doctors actually had his hand inside my belly, and it did not feel good at all. I remember feeling so bewildered wondering what they were doing to me. Just like a dream, I was suddenly in a situation that I couldn't understand. I was so upset and confused. It took a long time after I was off of pain medications before I could really understand the extent of what had happened to me. I am fortunate to remember as much of the experience as I do considering the circumstances I was experiencing.

Michelle was exhausted, sleeping a few hours here and there on the chair or couch in the ICU waiting room. She stayed at the hospital for the first four days, and was fortunate to be able to shower at the hospital in one of the resident's call rooms. I can't say enough about the incredible job the residents did bringing food, giving updates, and trying to help in any way that they could. The rotating persons who were taking care of Taylor and Chase did bring them to the hospital to see Michelle, but they did not take them in to see me for fear of truly scaring them. Michelle was so focused on me. Fortunately, our friends and family were able to pick up the slack with our other commitments. Later in the week, they convinced Michelle to go home for some brief visits. The large majority of her time was spent with me in the University Hospitals ICU.

Journal Entry 4/28/00

Good Morning Craig. Michelle and I got in around 6:30 am after her first night at home. We still had a hard time getting her to bed before 12:00, but at least she got more sleep, a shower and time to play with the boys. She's been a real trooper while trying to juggle the boys, house, news, pregnancy and being here with you.

John had a great time playing with the boys at the hospital. There are so many similarities with D and J. They played hide-n-seek, "can't get me" and gave John a tour of the hospital hot spots. John and I both wish our families were closer and could get together more often.

We are praying for you to be able to play with them again soon. Amy C.

By the next weekend, the various problems I was having seemed to have peaked and I was finally showing some slow improvement. With the difficulty in properly caring for my wounds, and knowing that I would need significant grafting and reconstruction, the ICU team worked steadily towards my stabilization so that I could be transferred to a facility which would be able to better accomplish these needs. My lungs had improved somewhat, and the ventilator settings had been backed down. My creatinine was slowly recovering, and though not at a normal level it was obvious that my kidneys were functioning better. My blood pressure had improved, although still requiring pressors to maintain it. I was still having fevers as different organisms saw their chance and were aggressively attacking me through my wounds. None were as life-threatening as the infection that started everything. I had gone back to the operating room several times for minor debridements, infected tissue removal, but not anywhere near to the extent of the surgery that had been done before. I had a few skin spots pop-up in random places, potential sites for more flesh-eating bacteria, but they had all been controlled with the minor debridements.

One moment of humor in the midst of all the stress was when the nurses decided I needed a shave. They had talked to Michelle about doing it. I was starting to look pretty scruffy but they had waited until there was some stability in my condition. Late in the week, they finally shaved me. Michelle couldn't help but laugh when she walked in and saw me. The nurses had left a mustache, and I guess it was quite a surprise. For some reason, the nurses thought that I normally wore a mustache, but they were mistaken. I guess it was not a good look for me. I have never been allowed to have facial hair of any consequence and that was fine from my standpoint. The beard and mustache issue would continue to be an issue throughout my illness. Even in my weakened state, my whiskers kept growing.

Journal Entry 4/29/00

Crash (my medical school nickname):

Today-the last 24 hours-has been one of great improvements. Creatinine down from a peak of 3.1 to 1.2; vent settings down from 100%, 10 peep AC24 to 40%; 5 peep and there's talk of weaning trials soon. Physically you are coming back to us-swelling receding rapidly-today knuckles and skin wrinkles returning. The mood is very positive though "cautiously optimistic" remains the prevailing undertone, you were so sick four days ago. G$ has been in contact at least daily and Lee too-I am grateful that my program let me come-it's hard to imagine the anticipation they have for any news-I will know it after tomorrow but don't like it. Among your physicians the mood is hopeful and initial talk of the "next step" appears to be in the early stages.

Craig, my family's prayers and thoughts are with you always-we love you and need you as part of our lives-and eagerly await our next "families" reunion. When in the greatest scheme you measure yourself as a man, physician, friend, etc.-the yardstick is how you have touched/affected the lives of those around you. I hope that in my life I at some point achieve a portion of the success that you have-you know and I know the reasons our bond is what it is-but the breadth and depth and volume of support by innumerable colleagues and friends poignantly demonstrates that you bless all the lives you touch-just as you have mine for some 7 years. As I grudgingly prepare to leave tomorrow morning, I want to quote one of my dearest friends on what was one of the toughest days of my life. While in a huge comforting hug he said to me, "I wish you were going with us....and I know you'll get everything you want." May flights of angels speed thy way.

All my love-your friend John C

Several close relationships developed between Michelle and the people taking care of me. Dr. Goldstein was so wonderful, frequently going out of his way to take time to talk with my family, even when he was utterly exhausted. He stayed at the hospital 24 hours a day for the first four days of my illness, only catching a few hours of sleep in his office when he could. My care was so labor-intensive with the dressing changes and debridements it was pointless for him to go home. I know this must have been incredibly hard on his family to have him so close but not home. Michelle also got to know several of the ICU nurses who frequently took care of me. Those medical professionals who invest themselves in relationships with their patients and families really can help by taking some of the burden of their patient's illness onto themselves. In the ten days I was in University Hospital's intensive care unit, I was fortunate enough to be cared for by several of these people, doctors and nurses willing to feel our pain as they helped us through such a difficult time. Hopefully, the way my family and friends pulled together behind me was in turn a good example for them, an example of true caring and support.

Journal Entries 4/30/00

I have meant to write in here all week - each of the day's events, concerns, blessings, etc., but I have either been too worried about you to concentrate, or too busy talking with all the visitors that have been here with us. Yesterday was a hard day for me, my spirits were low. Everything was looking better but your temperature was at its highest, 39.8 degrees C, and it was concerning me a lot. We had a family meeting yesterday with Dr. Goldstein to discuss "where to go from here." They discovered a yeast infection in your sputum, lungs and skin and are treating it with Diflucan, hoping that is what is contributing to your fever. I was sad for you and missed you an awful lot. But after talking with Dr. Goldstein, John C., John H. and ultimately Laurel I felt better about your fever and not so worried.

I went home again last night and slept on the couch from 12:20-6:10 and had the most sleep I have had since all of this started last Friday night. I had only been averaging four hrs. a night - I'll continue later-going in to see you. M-

Slick (another nickname):

We came yesterday, Saturday, but it was so disturbing to see you struggling to breathe, that I couldn't think of writing. What a difference a day makes. You look so much better today as does Michelle. We can see both of you are well-blessed with a strong faith, a caring family and wonderful friends. We've been impressed with all the expertise and TLC of the residents. Hang in there. A wonderful world awaits you and your family. All of you are surrounded by love and friends.

Linda

Hi Craig!

You probably don't know me and probably never will but I have taken care of you these last few days. You have made great strides these last couple of days and I have been there through it all. Your family is so supportive of you. I almost think that their strength in you could not fail in making you better. I would like to think it is my care but I know it is your will to live-to see your kids, family, etc. Good luck in these next few weeks! Get better soon!

Sincerely-
Lisa C, RN   MSICU-UH

Chapter 5

Helicopter Ride

Joshua 1:9 "Have I not commanded you? Be strong and courageous. Do not be terrified; do not be discouraged, for the Lord your God will be with you wherever you go."

Journal Entry - 5/1/00 @ 0300

Craig-

I don't know if you'll remember me, I cared for you the first four nights you spent in the MSICU and now the last night you'll be here since you'll transfer to Metrohealth tomorrow. Michelle was nice enough to request that I care for you so I could see you one last time before you transfer. You have an amazing wife, I have never seen anyone so devoted and in love. I hope to share the kind of bond you two have. I wish you all the luck in the world and hope you know what it has meant to care for you this week. You've given me more in faith, strength, and hope than I've given you in medical care. During the first days when you were still coherent, your questions were always about your wife and the baby, always making sure those around you were alright despite your condition. Come back and see us so we can see you without all the tubes! Good luck Craig!

Kristen, RN

Transferring patients between medical facilities is a relatively common occurrence in the United States. These transfers can occur for several reasons, including insurance and the need for more intensive or specialized care than the patient's original facility can provide. This was what happened in my case, I needed specialized wound care that would be best provided in a burn center. My clinical condition had improved quite a bit but I was far from being out of danger. I was still on a ventilator and being supported with fluids, blood, and pressors. I continued on multiple antibiotics and had intermittent high fevers. From my surgeries, I had lost about 30% of my skin surface along with large amounts of underlying muscle, leaving me with huge open wounds. My nutrition was being delivered through a tube in my nose down to my stomach. I was far from a picture of health.

Despite my devastated condition, my survival to this point was a miracle and everyone involved with my case was thankful for it. Was I stable enough to transfer to the burn unit? Though less than ten miles away, no one knew how I would respond to the stress of being moved. The decision-making process in regards to patient transfers is based on a risk-reward comparison. There are always risks involved with transfers, from the chance of an ambulance or helicopter accident to rapid de-stabilization during the trip. There are also several medical situations that shouldn't occur in the back of an ambulance or in a medical-evacuation helicopter. A prime example is a woman in premature labor. If there's any chance that the baby will be delivered during the transfer, it is preferable to have the baby delivered and then transferred rather than being born en route to the referral center. Once the reward of improved care outweighs the risks, it makes sense to transfer the patient to a place where they can receive the necessary care.

In my case, the big impetus to transfer was my wound care. This care was extremely labor-intensive, especially without any special wound care facilities at University Hospitals. There was also a finite period of time that my wounds could be "open" before major infection would set in, getting them covered with skin grafts sooner rather than later was a necessary goal. The burn unit at Metrohealth Hospital was the best place for my ongoing care for both reasons. The team debated sending me by ground or by air, and after much discussion, it was decided that the quicker ride in a helicopter would be better than the longer, bumpier ride in an ambulance. Dr. Goldstein had been in contact with Dr. Fratianne and Dr. Yowler from the burn unit at Metrohealth hospital, and they would accept me as a transfer once Dr. Goldstein and the ICU staff felt I was stable enough to make the trip.

No one knew how I would respond, yet, the transfer date was set for May 1st, assuming I would remain medically stable to that point. Since my condition had been so guarded during the majority of my ICU stay, the mention of transfer was only discussed with my family two days before it happened. The talk up to that stage had been about survival, my long-term needs were irrelevant if I didn't make it. Since this was such a new idea, my family had very mixed emotions about transferring. There were positive thoughts resulting from the fact that I was finally stable enough to move. There were also nervous thoughts about leaving their "comfort" zone and heading to a different hospital on the other side of town. In addition, there was the fear to move me in my fragile condition, and the fear of the helicopter ride itself. After receiving almost royal treatment at University Hospitals, it was hard to imagine starting over with new doctors, nurses and support staff, and without the overwhelming presence of those at Rainbow.

The morning of May 1st was a bright, sunny day, with little in the way of clouds. Weather can be a complicating factor in medical transfers, especially for helicopter travel. Wind, rain, fog, snow, sleet and ice all make flying in a helicopter much more treacherous. We were fortunate to not have the weather as a worry. After rounds by the ICU team and Dr. Goldstein in the morning, the decision to proceed with my transfer was made. Michelle and my mom were there. My dad was there but left in an attempt to get Taylor and Chase, hoping they might be able to see me takeoff in the helicopter. Unfortunately, a few wrong turns kept my dad and the boys from making it back to University Hospitals before I left. A flight team and helicopter from Metro arrived mid-morning and began assessing the situation. Michelle and my mom were very anxious as they watched the Metro team and the University Hospital's nurses unhook me from all my support mechanisms and rehook me to the portable equipment the crew had brought in from the helicopter. Would they hook up everything right? Everyone had to have faith that all the monitors and support devices would be attached correctly and I would not be left without anything vital. Being from a different hospital, the flight crew and the staff at Metro used some different equipment, so the transfer of all the tubes and wires was very tedious. The last thing to be detached was my ventilator. My breathing had to be maintained by one person squeezing an oxygen bag attached to my breathing tube for each breath I needed. This was more than my mom could bear to watch. She always struggled watching any of my breathing difficulties, so when they started bagging me, she excused herself. Michelle stayed for the last few minutes as they double-checked everything. She gave me a kiss and I was whisked away, down the back elevator to the waiting helicopter.

I had always wanted to take helicopter ride, but I don't remember anything about this trip. After about an hour of preparation, the helicopter air-time was only about 2 minutes. I guess that went fine, I never heard any more stories about the trip itself, although I'm sure that everyone involved was relieved once I was in the burn unit and back on a stationary ventilator.

What an overwhelming case I must have presented to the staff of doctors and nurses at Metro. Not that they couldn't handle it, but I was certainly a lot to take in. My nurse on that first day was AnnMarie. Later, she often talked about how sick I really was on arrival. My urine output that day had been very poor and all the stress of transfer had caused me to become clinically dehydrated. I was still quite feverish and I needed increased support from the ventilator. My wounds continued to leak tremendous amounts of fluid. As Michelle, my mom and later my dad, and Michelle's parents made the trip over to Metro, they had to wait several hours while the medical team assessed my condition and attempted to correct the deterioration I'd undergone during the trip. This was a very difficult time for my family. They were relieved once they were allowed to see me. The transfer had been completed without any real hitches, although it caused somewhat of a setback in my condition. No irreparable damage had occurred and now I was in the best facility to care for my wounds and reconstruct me. Being a patient in the burn unit would be a whole new experience as I entered a new phase of my recovery.

Journal Entry - 5/1/00

At about 11:45 am I left you to be brought to Metro by helicopter. I was very nervous! The transport went well but your blood pressure dropped into the 70's and you stopped urinating. But as the day went on they were able to push you with fluids to help both functions improve. You still had a very high fever, 104-105 degrees. They were able to come down on the vent to 40% Oxygen as well.

M-

Chapter 6

Burn Unit

The transition of my care from University Hospitals to Metrohealth Hospital was initially difficult and stressful for my family. I was at a new hospital on the other side of town, without all the support of everyone from my residency program. Michelle went from semi-VIP status at University Hospitals to just another family member at Metro, which was frustrating for her, as it would be for anyone in her situation. She was used to being given information on a minute-by-minute basis, but the team at Metro didn't do things that way. While the ICU at University Hospitals had rules, the burn unit at Metro was much more rigid in structure and regulations, for good reason. These strict regulations are aimed at decreasing the likelihood of infection, one of the most feared complications for burn victims. There were restrictions at University Hospitals ICU, but not to the extent of those at the burn unit. Michelle, wanting to be so involved and not being familiar with their protocol, felt like she was being kept out of my care more than before. Once the people at Metro understood her need for constant information and involvement in my care, they were able to work with her and build good relationships. Building these good ties with new physicians, nurses and staff took time, and was worth all the effort in making my difficult situation as positive as possible.

Journal Entry - 5/2/00

It is quite an abrupt change being here instead of at UH. We are thankful you are here for the expert, proper care but it has been a change for us to get to know everyone new, the new rules, hospital, and lack of being able to keep in touch with others well, not getting explanation of medical terms that are confusing as much, etc. Today you look good - urine better, creatinine at 2.0 now, pressure in the low 100's to 110's, vent at 30% O2, but you are still very hot. Your dressing change went well this morning the nurses and music therapist said. They are also concerned that you aren't waking up as much as you should be, so they have sent you for some tests - CT scan of your head, sinuses and abdomen, and a test for your adrenal-gland function so maybe we can get some answers. We saw you wheeled by and back. CT scan you did fine with; we are awaiting the results. A social worker came to see us and Mr. R. from pastoral care came to talk with us.

We are **so** thankful - the news is encouraging! No internal bleeding anywhere! They did find some fluid in your right mastoid that ENT will come look at more closely for infection. We will have to wait until tomorrow to find out the results of the adrenal gland test, but they did say they will start you on some steroids.

I went in to visit you and ENT (ear, nose and throat) and ID (infectious disease) were there and talked with me at length. ENT doesn't think the mastoid is infected, but they did find drainage in your left ear that they will culture. ID just talked with me about the antibiotics you are on and their rationale. Dr. Goldstein called me too and seemed pleased about your progress for the day too. Fever down some in the 38's (around 101 F), creatinine to 1.6, blood pressure about the same, vent at 30%. Your dad, my mom and me today, John H. came by. M-

Over the next few days, my condition slowly improved, yet I was still pretty out of it and continued to require a breathing tube. The multiple antibiotics were continuing as did the fevers. As often happens after being in the hospital for an extended period of time, I began to get other "opportunistic" infections, meaning that when my defenses were down, these micro-organisms took advantage and caused infection. These infections caused my daily fevers and needed to be controlled for any skin grafting to work. On a good note, my edema, the extra fluid in my tissues was subsiding. Prior to my illness I averaged around 200 lbs., then I ballooned to 250 lbs. from all the fluid and now my weight was falling on the way to a low of under 150 lbs. All of my muscles were atrophying, wasting away, due to my lack of movement and muscle use. Nutrition, started at University Hospitals and continued at Metro, was pumped through a tube in my nose at an incredible 4000 calories a day, but even that could not provide the needed calories to maintain my weight, fight the infection and heal. Burn victims and anyone with large skin and tissue loss require incredible amounts of calories to heal. Apparently, it was quite a drastic change in how I looked, losing 100 lbs. in the matter of a few weeks.

Journal Entry 5/4/00

Hi Punkin! Well, you look good today, another day to Praise the Lord! Your temp is actually a bit low today at 36.6, no more fever and the dressing change cooled you off some, HR in low 90's, pressure 130/50, so more stable overall, vent same only tidal volume increased to 700 from 650. Wounds look great and ready for surgery tomorrow. You are still acidotic and would like to get that under more control, so they have changed some things. I can't remember the word she used. Can't wait to speak to the doctor about tomorrow. We're getting to know people here better now, so that is helping our comfort level. The boys really miss you - Taylor cried yesterday when we left. My mom said he couldn't understand why he couldn't come to see you too. Then this morning Chase asked for you again and I asked him if he missed you, he said yes. Then at night when I get home he tells me "I cried for you mommy." It's hard wanting to be everything for all of you and not being able to, but we're managing, taking one day at a time. Thank the Lord for both sets of parents! My parents do have to go back Sunday for the work week and then will be back on the weekend again. Your dad hasn't made any decisions yet - depends on you, and your mom is staying since school for her is out and I could really use her help. I love you baby so much! You did try to open your eyes a bit for me today - nice to know you recognized my voice. M-

To deal with the problem of my large skin defects, Drs. Fratianne and Yowler made the decision to use pig skin to cover these areas, with two goals in mind. First, it would act as a barrier for infection, even if only temporarily, and secondly, it would give the doctors an idea if my body was to the point to be able to accept skin grafts from my own healthy skin. The pig skin was put in place with staples in the operating room. Unfortunately, this first application was only about fifty percent successful. The pig skin graft failed to take at all on my back, while it did take on several areas of my front. The pig skin that didn't take was removed or fell off. With the emotional rollercoaster that everyone was riding, this setback was very disheartening for my family. As each hurdle during my illness approached, the anticipation heightened with the stakes. My failure to overcome any of these hurdles could result in complications and ultimately my death, so setbacks of any type were hard to take. The failure of the first pig skin application was a clear sign that I wasn't ready for my actual skin-grafting. My family knew that I had a small window of time to get grafted, so while this failure wasn't fatal, the clock was ticking and everyone knew it. The defects needed to be closed before infections of my wounds became overwhelming.

Journal Entry - 5/8/00

Yesterday looked very promising - no fever, all other vitals real good and the nurse said what she could see of the pig skin looked real good. But today my heart is heavy for you again. I haven't cried in a few days (much at least), but today it all feels like draining out. I still have to keep the faith and hope that this is just a delay and you and the Lord will prevail! Some days are easier than others (you're well = I'm well and vice-versa). Today Dr. Yowler looked at your pig skin grafts and we had half and half news. Your back didn't take at all, but 85% of the front did. Of course I always hope for things to work out perfectly, and then I get reminded that it is not an easy road we are traveling here - there are many bumps on the way. They did say that there is also a fungus on your back, so will be treating you with Nystatin cream beginning tomorrow. They also hope to get you weaned off the vent by Wednesday or Thursday of this week. I would feel better with that endotracheal tube out of you to decrease the chance of infection. As a bonus, you would be happier and then you could talk to us as well. Oh - one day at a time.

I hope you don't find this silly or boring to read later, it just is an easier way to remember each day (for you later) and it is the only way I can "tell" you my feelings now. I do tell you verbally - I talk with you, pray with you, play CD's for you and touch your arms, hands, face and hair daily, hoping subconsciously you can feel me here with you. Oh how I do miss you baby and just pray so hard each day - many, many times that this will all continue to go in a positive direction and we will enjoy one another again and the many dreams in life ahead of us. God is good, I know that, and I know that he is in control of all of this and holds you each day (wish I could!) in his loving arms.

Well I am going to go back in now and sit with you some more since that __is__ what I am here to do. Love you babe, with all I am and have! M-

As we went through this first week in the burn unit, Michelle describes me as being mostly asleep, but opening my eyes at times and acknowledging the people around me. I remember this time as well, but my remembrances are very abstract. Still to this day, I can look back and remember a lot of the visions or dreams I had as they were so vivid. I also remember how none of the situations I found myself in made sense to me. The drugs I had been given for pain and sedation such as Ativan and Morphine had really taken their toll on my perceptions. The encouraging part for others going through the similar experience of a drug-induced coma was that I had many "dreams" that included lots of those people who visited me. Almost as an "out of body" experience, I never could understand what was happening to me. I couldn't seem to do what I wanted, but I definitely interacted with family, nurses and doctors during this drug-clouded state. The talking, visiting and interacting with patients in these drug-induced states is extremely worthwhile and should be encouraged. Even if patients don't respond or respond inappropriately, they still indirectly know that you're there for them. All the settings that I found myself in are almost comical to think about now. Sometimes, they were places I had been before and sometimes they seemed totally abstract. Almost every dream had a common thread running through it, that I was somehow being held against my will. I remember feeling pain and trying hard to change what was happening to me in these dreams, but was always unsuccessful. I don't know what the people around me were seeing me do while I was having these dreams, but from the sounds of things after about three weeks, I was occasionally alert enough to make eye contact with those around me.

My most vivid dreams were about being bathed. These were not normal baths, but were strangely painful and irritating. I couldn't understand why the people helping me bathe were hurting me so much. Looking back, I'm sure these dreams corresponded with trips to the spray table, but again I didn't know what was going on at the time. My dreams included some of the people who came to visit in the hospital, but not all. Why this is I'll never know, perhaps I did dream about them and have just lost the recollection of them.

It was about this time that something special arrived in the mail. We had actually been flooded with cards from well-wishers from all over the country, but this was a bigger, soft package. Michelle said she was so confused, it had a return address from Penn State Athletics. As she opened it up, she just burst into tears. Inside the package was a Penn State football jersey with my old number, 49, on it. Included was a letter from Joe Paterno himself. It read:

May 4, 2000

Dear Craig:
I understand you have had some serious health problems and am pleased to get the report that you are improving. I am sorry about the problems you encountered. Hang in there and keep your chin up.

I am sending you a jersey to give you some extra incentive to get well quickly. With the changes in our coaching staff, the challenging Big Ten schedule, and the inexperience of our team, we may need you to "suit up" for this year. Of course, I will have to check to see if you have any remaining eligibility! Seriously, Craig, take care of yourself and I hope the next report I get about you is that you have fully recovered from this setback.

Best wishes and regards.
Sincerely,
Joe P

As Michelle shared this with both of our parents, I guess everyone had a good cry around the kitchen table. The word of my illness had even spread to my former college football coach in Pennsylvania. It was pretty amazing to me that Coach Paterno would take the time to write and send a jersey to me, a walk-on who had never contributed much to the program. That is just the kind of man he is. It meant so much to my family, they even put the letter in a frame and brought it in to my room in the burn unit. It certainly made a good conversation piece for all my visitors. I wasn't awake to enjoy it at this point but was pleasantly surprised when I was awake enough to hear about it. By the way, I do still have some eligibility remaining but I don't plan on ever using it. The coaches are glad for that.

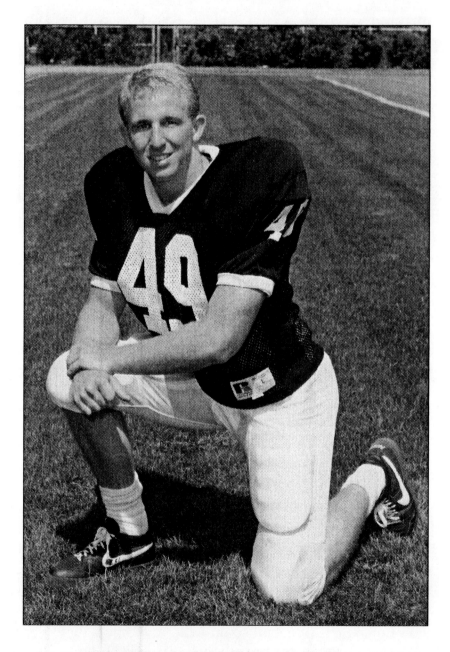

A 1988 picture of Craig in uniform as a
freshman football player at Penn State.

This time after my first pig skin application was one of great impatience. Things were better now almost three weeks into this ordeal, but I still had to get my wounds covered, my fevers under control and my breathing to the point where I could come off of the ventilator. As is often the case in any critical care situation, yet another problem developed. I had developed deep venous thromboses, DVT's, in both of my legs from lying still in bed for so long. This is unfortunately a very common occurrence in anyone critically ill or anyone immobilized for an extended period of time. To treat this I was placed on a medicine called heparin as a continuous drip into my IV. Heparin is a drug to keep your blood thin and prevent more clots from being produced. Clots in blood vessels can lead to problems around the site of the clot, infection and/or inflammation in the surrounding tissue known as phlebitis. Even more serious is the possibility of a pulmonary embolus. This means that part or all of the clots are loosed, leaving the site in the leg and traveling through the right side of the heart and lodging in the lungs. Depending on the site and size of the clot, this can be extremely serious and even fatal. While not a guaranteed preventative measure, treating with the heparin is very good at preventing this from occurring. As if we needed another problem to worry about, this problem was added to my long list!

Trying again, a second application of pig skin was put on my open wounds three days after the first attempt. This time could also be characterized as a limited success with the majority of difficulties still being found on my back. There was some concern that a yeast infection had taken over my wounds there and any grafting wouldn't be successful until that was well treated. Despite being on two high-power antibiotics and one high-power antifungal, I continued to have daily fevers. My white blood-cell count was about 32, normal being 6 to 12, so these high counts were making all of my doctors nervous. Some of the physicians who were working with me believed that the high WBC count was due to the steroids I was being given for my adrenal suppression. The high white blood-cell count is a well-known side effect of steroid treatment, but with my fevers continuing daily, the concern for worsening infection was ever-present and on everyone's mind.

Meanwhile, my breathing had become stronger and stronger, and the day after my second pigskin application, May 11, I was finally extubated. Being extubated meant the breathing tube was pulled out and kept out for the first time since this ordeal started. What a relief it was for me to be able to breathe on my own again. It was not easy to deal with all the secretions I had in my throat and mouth, but I was so glad to have that tube out. The nurses kept a suction device right at my bed to continuously remove these secretions as I coughed them up. Michelle, other family members or the nurses had the almost constant job of sucking out my mouth as mucus seemed to be continuously appearing. I was too weak at this point to do it for myself. Anyone who has ever been awake with a breathing tube in your throat knows that it is one of the most uncomfortable and terrifying feelings possible. The constant gagging pressure of what feels like a garden hose in your throat, coupled with the inability to make a sound leaves you feeling vulnerable, crazy, helpless and desperate to get that tube out. It is no wonder that lots of sedation is used for patients who are intubated to keep them from pulling out their tube or going insane. So, after several days of being awake enough to be miserable with the tube in, the tube was finally out. This was such a milestone for me in terms of comfort. I was able to communicate and the doctors were finally able to significantly reduce the pain medications because the breathing tube was no longer an issue. As a result, I was a little more clear-headed and better able to interact with family and friends that came to visit.

Journal Entry - 5/11/00

We got here about 9:30 AM this morning (your dad and I). Praise the Lord!!! We just got the news - you have been extubated! (10:10

50

AM) What a great accomplishment for you today. Now I just want to hear that your white count has dropped too and I'll feel great - I'm probably asking too much but I just want so much for you baby! The Lord truly has blessed us all! I cannot wait to see you sweetheart - wish I was in there right now. I just can't even put my feelings for you into words right now. I just wish I could hold you - there will be a day I can - I'll just be patient. M

5/12/00

I am sorry I didn't get to write much yesterday, but I was in with you the whole day except to eat lunch and dinner as quickly as I could. You did really well coming off the vent yesterday - you are so strong! You went from 100 percent oxygen to 28 percent oxygen and from the mask to the nasal cannula without any problems - sats good, blood gases good. All your vitals were good too. They took you off the ativan and morphine completely for a bit while extubating you to help you wake up some more. But then Dr. Kwan (a resident physician in the Burn Unit) wanted you to respond pretty quick I thought. Everyone had been saying you are on such high doses of sedation it would take awhile and then they seem to expect you to come out of it pretty quick. I understand why - they wanted you to be able to protect your airway, especially since you had so many thick secretions in your lungs when they pulled the tube out. They were contemplating having to put it back in, but were greatly encouraged when they saw you cough for awhile, and answer a few questions. As the day went on, you were able to respond more, keep your eyes opened (not focused very well yet) and answer some questions. Understandably so you are also very tired too. The nurse during the night asked you which CD you wanted her to put on -Lynyrd Skynyrd and she said you opened your eyes and nodded yes! And seemed a bit excited. So they were sure to play that while you were being extubated! It was nice to see you try to open your eyes and smile at me twice yesterday - my heart just melted! I sure do love you sweetheart. I'm anxious to see you today. I would have stayed the night with you, but I had to check with the head nurse. So I'll ask. I hated to leave you last night. I'm sure you're still so confused about what is going on and have so many questions. I wish I could just know you're thinking and your comprehension capabilities. I know you to have a sore throat and have so much junk and that it is difficult for you to talk, even if you want to - poor guy. I got a chart today and maybe I can point to it and you can blink if it is something you want or maybe can point to it yourself. Well, I can go back to see you now, so continue later. Love you. M-

I still had not seen my boys during my entire illness. With the help of the social workers and child-life specialists, it had been determined that it was better to wait until I was in a little better condition before letting them see me. Now, being more awake and having my breathing tube out, we began making preparations for them to see me.

The next several days were good ones, getting caught up with family and friends and learning more about what had really happened to me. I was pretty confused and at one point I even asked Michelle if I had totaled my car in an accident. I had a recurring vision of a tractor-trailer carrying gasoline crushing into me on the Innerbelt bridge in Cleveland. I even know the company name on the truck. It took a while for the truth about what happened to me since I'd gone into the hospital back on April 22nd to truly sink in. This was a very emotional time for me as well. As the pieces of everything that had occurred started coming together, the realization of what had happened and what was to come really hit home with me. I remember Dr. Fratianne telling me that it would be Christmas before I felt somewhat back to normal. I was devastated, I had so much to do prior to Christmas, there was no way I could delay things that long. In retrospect he was right on, I did do lots of things before Christmas but I didn't begin to feel "normal" until well after Christmas.

Journal Entry - 5/14/00

Hi sweetheart. I came in with both of my parents this morning to see you and stayed until only one o'clock. Then I went home to have lunch with everyone for the first time since we've all been together. Keith had sent some ribs to your mom for Mother's Day, so she made these and a really nice big lunch with strawberry shortcake for dessert. It was nice, but I hated to have to leave you for that. I am back (3:40) and Bridget, your nurse said they are going to try to put you in the cardiac chair, so would be a half an hour until you'd be situated for us to come back. So I decided it would be a good time to write.

You look really good today and are more awake. You talked with me, ate ice chips and a grape popsicle and respiratory was in to give you your deep-breathing treatment for about 30 minutes total. It was nice. I feel bad though because I can't understand your raspy whispers very well. You try so hard and I can't understand - how frustrating for you. I am sorry. You are still coughing up stuff and I've been helping suction it out. I wish I could do more for you though. Each day will be better. They have tentatively scheduled your surgery for your belly skin grafts to be done on Wednesday. Everyone keeps saying how good your wounds look, so that is encouraging. Well, time to go and see how the chair is working out. Love you!

Wow! You looked great sitting up and awake. We talked and fed you ice chips for one hour and 10 minutes before you fell asleep. You asked about so many things - things that are supposed to happen in the future. You asked me to take the splint on your arm off because it felt like your two fingers were sticking together. You got emotional at one point after we told you who was here to see you, who has called, etc. A lot for you to take in and handle at once I know. I told you that we all have had three weeks to cry, worry, pray, etc. and that it would take some time for you to and that you're allowed to feel! I hope you do baby - and talk to me about everything you want, whenever you want (confidentially, I promise). I want to always be there for you in any way I can. We're best friends and you're everything to me. I'm so thankful to *still have you - what a blessing you are to me. I thank God daily and for all He has done for you and me through this trauma.*

Philippians 4: 8 "finally brothers, whatever is true, whatever is noble, whatever is right, whatever is pure, whatever is lovely, whatever is admirable - if anything is excellent or praiseworthy think about such things."*

M-

Not long after I was awake and talking again, I was visited by Dr. Nieder, my residency program director; Dr. Avner, the department head of pediatrics at Rainbow; and Dr. Lorentz, one of our chief residents. For them to take the time to drive across town to see me meant a lot. I was nervous about them coming, in some ways I didn't want them to see me looking so bad, but otherwise I was glad to have them come. I raised the head of my bed as far as I could stand it and made sure my hair was washed. I also had the nurses shave me. I'm sure I still looked terrible, but I put my best face on. I felt bad for them because everyone had to wear masks, gowns and gloves while in my room. It gave me the sense that I had the plague, but actually it was my visitors germs they were trying to keep away from me. My visitors were uncomfortably hot as a result, the plastic didn't breathe very well. I asked frequently for my room to be cooler, but I was usually told that it was against the rules. Dressed in only a hospital gown, when I got hot or feverish, I could only get uncovered to cool off. That strategy didn't work well with visitors coming in. I had lost any sense of modesty but I usually made an effort to keep myself covered when others were around.

The visit by the group from Rainbow went well and picked me up a little. I told them as much as I could about the future surgeries I was to have and they let me know about the happenings at Rainbow. They also let me know what they had worked out for me in terms of finishing my residency. Because of elective and basic requirements, I had to complete one more month doing a behavioral rotation to meet national standards. In one sense, the timing of my illness was good in that all of my difficult on-call months had already been completed. If I had needed to do any months with overnight call, we would have been stuck in Cleveland much longer in order for me to get rehabilitated enough to make it through a 36 hour shift. Looking back, that could have extended our stay by six months or more. The doctors' and everyone else from Rainbow's efforts to see me and support me and my family through all of our struggles were so appreciated. I couldn't have been more fortunate in this regard.

Just as things seemed to be looking up, another complication developed. One night, I began vomiting large amounts of bright, red blood. This happened when I grabbed my feeding tube and pulled it out of my nose. I don't remember pulling it out, so I'm not sure if it was accidental or purposeful. I do have a vague recollection of vomiting up the blood, but even that is very fuzzy. Though it seemed to be a one-time occurence, I later underwent an endoscopy to make sure there weren't any spots inside my esophagus or stomach that would be a source for such bleeding. An endoscopy is a procedure where a small camera is passed through the mouth down into the stomach to look at its lining. The instrument can even take small biopsies if needed. The endoscopy occurred a few days later, and unfortunately I remember every minute of that procedure. Because I had already been on so much pain medication, they were unable to put me to sleep until long after the procedure was over. I watched the monitor along with the doctors as the probe looked at all the lining of my esophagus and stomach. Since my endoscopy was basically normal with just one small possible ulcer, the bleeding was thought to be caused by my heparin therapy. I still had clots in my legs but was having trouble with the heparin, so the decision was made to place a filter in my inferior vena cava, the large vein that drains the entire body into the right side of the heart.

This screen serves as a blocker should any of the clots in my leg come loose. The clots would be prevented from passing through my heart up into my lungs. This filter remains in me to this day, and to this point has done its job protecting me from clots going to my lungs. Once the filter was in place and my lungs were protected, the doctors stopped the heparin to try to prevent any more bleeding from my GI tract.

Journal Entry - 5/15/00

Joshua 1:9 *"Have I'm not commanded you? Be strong and courageous. Do not be terrified; do not be discouraged, for the Lord your God will be with you wherever you go."*

I looked this up this morning because I was feeling discouraged by your morning update. I spoke with the resident on-call and she told me about your night. At 2:00 AM you threw up some blood. You had ripped out your feeding tube and as they tried to put it back in you threw up. So, seeing blood, they put in a new NG tube and flushed you out with six ounces of water. They did not see any fresh blood, but only old blood, which is good. They still had to stop your heparin because of possible internal bleeding, therefore it is necessary to put a screen in your groin to keep the clots in your leg from going up to your lungs. They talked about scoping your stomach for an ulcer or stress ulcer, but we haven't talked with the Dr. yet, so we'll see. Dr. Fratianne begins service today for two weeks, so we'll get to meet him for the first time. He is supposed to come and talk with us after your dressing change - which is going on right now. I was happy to hear you asked about me today. You are so cute. I just love you with all my heart babe. I'm having a rough day myself. I'm trying to figure out all this housing stuff too and it is so overwhelming. Chase cried when I left this morning too. And then being pregnant on top of that all does not help the emotions one bit - and you know me to begin with. It's lonely feeling this way. You're usually the shoulder I cry on, and I can't do that; I need to be strong for you too, to help you get through this. This is so hard, I know, but we will make it!

Well, Dr. Fratianne is so nice and just spoke with us calmly about everything. He said that he does think the heparin is what caused the bleeding and now with that off and the screen in, you should be fine. You are still scheduled for surgery on Wednesday, Dr. Fratianne seems to think that only the chest flaps will be ready and grafting any more will have to be determined at the time of the surgery when the pig skin comes off. Dr. Yowler will do that surgery on Wednesday and make those decisions. And Friday, it will be Dr. Frat's decision because he will cover you for a few weeks. So we will pray for the best. Glad it still looks like we're moving forward. M-

Now that my breathing tube was out, the date was set for my skin-grafting surgery. I got so nervous about it. It was so nice to be interacting with my family and friends, I had no desire to be put under again. On one hand, I just really wanted to get it over with, but I was also not looking forward to being intubated again. Just as I was starting to come out of my drugged state, the time for my grafting surgery arrived on May 17. The surgery took over six hours, but they were able to graft most of my wounds during that one procedure. There had been some concern that it would take two or more surgeries to be able to get all the work done, but I tolerated things well enough to get everything finished at once. What a blessing for me to have everything but my armpit grafted. The original plan had been to leave me intubated overnight so I could get some needed rest, but the balloon on my breathing tube actually popped, so they had to take it out that night. This was fine with me and my breathing actually went well without the tube.

The act of skin grafting is a very gruesome but lifesaving procedure that involves taking the top layers of skin from healthy skin elsewhere on the body and placing it over top of the defects. I had never seen it done prior to my experience, but I recently saw it on a program from the Discovery Health Channel. The surgeon takes an instrument that works similar to a wire cheese slicer to remove the desired thickness of skin. This skin is then laid over top of the defects and sutured and stapled into place. A special material is then placed over top of both the do-nor-sites and the graft-sites and stapled into place. I would venture to guess that I had over 1000 staples put into me and later removed, one by one. Once all the skin grafting was completed, I was wrapped in bandages from what seemed like head to toe. Except for my armpit, all the grafts were now in place, and everyone anxiously waited to see if they would take, or whether more grafting would be necessary.

After the big step of skin grafting was completed, the next phase of my illness could be characterized by one word, pain. This pain came mostly from the donor sites where the skin for my grafts had been taken. I had these donor sites in long strips on both legs, all the way around my thigh from my hip to just above my knee. I also had a few on the good side of my torso, side, and back, so from my chin to my knees, I was almost all graft and donor sites. Pressure, movement, air and moisture; all these caused my donor sites incredible pain. I felt like I'd been dragged naked across asphalt, leaving me with excruciating brush burns. As if the donor sites weren't bad enough, I still had a tube in my nose providing my nutrition. This tube caused me significant nausea and some intermittent vomiting. I was clothed in a "frat jacket," named in honor of my surgeon, Dr. Fratianne. This jacket was a conglomeration of all kinds of drains and bandages surrounding all the graft areas. This felt so tight that it seemed to constrict my breathing. All the fluids used to bathe my new grafts would pool in my bed. This resulted in having my bed changed multiple times everyday. Getting my bed changed was very aggravating and uncomfortable since I couldn't get up myself. I would be rolled around, while clean linens were jammed underneath me. I was alive, barely, but life in this state was awful. I can still remember thinking, how could this have happened to me? It was more disbelief than anger at this point. It was a hard existence, I was either asleep or in pain, there wasn't any other choice at that stage. Everyone around me was trying to be positive, hoping the grafts would take and my recovery could move forward.

Pain is unfortunately a very common component of any serious illness. From blood draws and IV line placements to more invasive procedures, pain is something that must be dealt with constantly. Along with procedures, the illness or injury itself can also be a cause of pain, and this is often the most difficult kind of pain to manage. The pain that we feel is composed of two distinct parts, both physical and emotional. Both areas need to be addressed for pain to be controlled as best as possible.

Pain was certainly a large part of my illness. The amount of pain medication I received over the two months I was hospitalized is staggering. For weeks, I was kept comfortable and mostly unconscious with massive amounts of medication. This medicating continued for all my post-surgical pain and daily torture sessions on the spray table. The difficult thing about pain medicines is that their effect decreases over time as the body is able to metabolize and breakdown these medicines more quickly. To reach the same amount of pain relief, increasing doses of pain medication are needed. By the end of my hospitalization, I was requiring huge doses of medicine to feel any relief. These doses would knock me out now. Everyone has their own personal feelings about using pain medications. Once I was making those decisions, my preference was to use as little as possible. It is a combination of the undesirable side effects from the medicines and my tough-guy feelings that make me view using pain medication as a last resort. Even with my feelings being what they are, I used lots of medicine during my illness. Everyone handles pain differently, so each case should be dealt with on an individual basis. Doctors also have to balance their patient's comfort with the potential detriment these medicines can do to their condition. Like a double-edged sword, pain medicines have an important role in decreasing pain but also have side effects that can slow recovery or rehabilitation.

I can still recall many episodes where the pain was so excruciating that it led me to tears. The worst time came on the spray table one day. The order must have come down from above that the materials covering the donor sites on my legs had to go. The nurses kept working even though I begged them to stop, pulling apart flesh and material that were trying hard to stay together. I pleaded with them to no avail, they kept going. The pain went to a level I don't believe I'd ever been to, other than at the start of my whole illness. I lost all control and started sobbing my guts out. I couldn't hear anything the nurses were saying to me, it was as if my brain removed itself from my body for a few minutes. I have read about people having similar feelings as they were tortured to this level. Fortunately, I never got to that point again throughout my illness.

Having experienced events like this, there were certainly times when the pain got to me emotionally. I would spend all my time worrying about my next trip to the spray table. It got so bad that I actually requested to have some donor site bandages removed during one of my follow-up operations while I was under general anesthesia . The intense pain from my donor sites lasted two weeks before starting to subside. Because I had multiple operations that included skin grafting, I had to go through this difficult two-week period several times. With the help of the pain medications, distractions, some attempts at controlled breathing, and very caring and understanding nurses, I was able to make it through the worst pain of my life. What other choice did I have?

Isaiah 40:28-31 "Do you not know? Have you not heard? The Lord is the everlasting God, the Creator of the ends of the earth. He will not grow tired and weary, and his understanding no one can fathom. He gives strength to the weary and increases the power of the weak. Even youths grow tired and weary, and young men stumble and fall; but those who hope in the Lord will renew their strength. They will soar on wings like eagles; they will run and not grow weary, they will walk and not be faint."

For four days after my grafting surgery the soaking and bed-changing cycle continued. Then the day of reckoning arrived, the day when the bandages would be removed and the grafts would be checked for the first time. Everyone was anxious to see how well they had taken. I wasn't sure what to expect, but it turned into a real experience for everyone involved. My physical therapist, Tami, was there. Her difficult job was to help me get into the necessary positions, enabling the staff to remove my bandages. The biggest difficulty I faced was that I didn't have the strength to sit up, so the doctors could look at the areas around my torso. I don't remember exactly how she got me into the sitting position, but I vividly remember semi-sitting on the edge of my hospital bed with Tami on her knees underneath me, supporting my weight so I didn't collapse onto the floor. Just the strain of that position was so incredibly painful and tiring. It left me feeling as if I couldn't breathe. The room was full of every available helper so it felt chaotic as orders were barked and my grafts were unwrapped, evaluated and re-bandaged as quickly as possible. While the discomfort of the procedure was awful, the result was well worth it. The grafts had taken well in eighty to ninety percent of the areas grafted. There was such a deep hole under my left shoulder blade where grafting had not even been attempted. The nurses were stuffing this hole with packing material daily which was also very unpleasant. It felt like they were stuffing the packing directly into my chest. The pain was dull and achy rather than sharp. This is due to the fact that the pain fibers inside our body work differently than those of our skin. All pain is very localized when things happen to the outside of us, it is a much more generalized, all-over, pain when it in occurs internally. Internal pain is just as uncomfortable as pain on the external surfaces, just in a different way. Dr. Fratianne and Dr. Yowler both were very pleased with the success of the grafting, and now that it was over, my rehabilitation and healing could progress.

One night, as Michelle and her parents were visiting me, the patient in the next room of the burn unit "coded." This word is medical jargon for an emergency, a sudden arrest of cardiorespiratory function. I was lying in bed, talking with Michelle and her parents, Stephen and Carolyn, when the alarms started sounding. Doctors and nurses were suddenly rushing down the hall yelling for help while the alarms continued to blare. Although I had been through many similar situations as a doctor, this event affected me much more personally as a patient. I started to feel funny, my heart started pounding, almost as if it was trying to jump out of my chest. I begin to shiver, getting colder and colder. In retrospect, I most likely was having a panic attack. I kept trying to calm myself, to think calming thoughts and not internalize the horrible event happening next door, but I couldn't control it. My body was reacting to an event and my mind was unable to control this reaction. To the best of my recollection, I have never had another episode like this and I hope that I never will. This was very scary for Michelle's parents as well, as it would be for anyone so close to such a terrible occurrence. Michelle and her dad piled on as many blankets as they could find to help my shivering cold. Carolyn decided to go back to the burn-unit waiting room as it was too upsetting. Although I had never met any of the other patients or their families, my family had met several of the family members of the patients in the burn unit. We did know what this particular patient was dealing with, so that made the whole situation more personal and devastating for us. After some time, one of the nurses came to check on me and noticed how I was reacting and gave me some medicine to calm down. I must have finally fallen asleep. The next morning I found out that the patient next door did not survive. It was easy to mentally put myself into the same situation. That could have been me dying. We all mourned for her. This event vividly reminded us of how fortunate we were to survive each critical step, and we couldn't take anything for granted.

Journal Entry - 5/20/00

Wow, I haven't found the time in two days to write in here. Sorry. A quick update on Thursday and Friday was that they changed one antibiotic to cover E.Coli and Pseudomonas, but that they weren't surprised to have them cultured - kind of expecting it I guess. Other than that, your vitals have been great and stable, urine output still good. But you've been nauseated for two days now and we couldn't make sense of why until last night when Dr. Kwan noticed your feeds are going into your stomach instead of further down like it should. Poor guy! So they did give you Reglan to help since you said the Compazine didn't seem to touch it. The nurse last night said she gave you some Ativan and Reglan and you seemed to sleep better. I was so relieved. You said you felt better at 5:30 AM, so I was very glad for you to have some relief from the nausea. Then you were taken in for your dressings to be looked at 7:15 AM. We arrived here (both moms and I) at 9:40 and Bonnie told us that you're grafts look good - about 90 percent taken!

Yes! God is so good! What a major praise. We are so thankful for you that the Lord seemed to lead the doctors to the right decision to graft everything and they look so good now. I will continue to pray that it stays that way until Monday. I was so worried about you last night when the 84-year-old lady next door to you coded and everyone went crazy trying to revive her. Your blood pressure, respirations and heart rate went sky high and it took awhile for you to relax and calm down. I hated to leave you. I came home when you got tired but I woke up at 1:30 and called to check on you. I could not get through until 2 o'clock, but I was relieved to hear you were given the Reglan and Ativan and were sleeping. She said you had a good night after that. M-

Now my days were filled with daily trips to the spray table, and therapy to increase the strength in my legs and shoulder. In between these activities, I would see visitors and catch naps. The nights were torture for me. It was impossible for me to sleep for long periods of time, so I slept here and there one to two hours at a time. This was due to many factors, my pain and uncomfortable positions, the pain medication, and the continued fevers which were always worse at night. Michelle, my parents, or whoever was visiting would usually leave me at 10 or 11 p.m., then I would sleep for an hour or two, usually wake up in a sweat, watch TV for an hour or two, and repeat the cycle through the night. I had never seen so much late-night TV. I usually awoke dreaming that I was running away from somebody or something. I was never quite sure, but woke up drenched in sweat and couldn't tell what was chasing me. I often felt nauseous when I awoke from these dreams. One night during this process I awoke with lots of attention. There were several nurses and a resident in the room with me. I didn't find this out until later but my heart-rate had dropped to a very slow rate, also known as a bradycardia. I'm still not sure why this happened, but it got everyone upset and concerned. Since it was quite significant, the doctors decided that my heart needed checked out. The normal way with an echocardiogram wasn't an option since I had fresh grafts right over my heart. I had to have a TEE, trans-esophageal echocardiogram, which meant I had to swallow the camera to look at my heart from the inside. It was another uncomfortable procedure where sedation didn't work. So, I simply endured having this tube down through my throat and into my esophagus. Fortunately, the results were good, no abnormalities were seen.

My sleep deprivation at night resulted in my taking several short naps during the day. I tried not to do this when visitors were around, but sometimes sleep would not be denied. I guess it was from my lack of energy from everything I had gone through, but I could fall asleep without even realizing it. This was uncharacteristic of me and fortunately everyone seemed to be understanding. The longest nap was always after my trip to the spray table. I was usually so exhausted, freezing cold, and medicated that my return almost always was followed by a two to three hour nap. The nurses would layer blankets over me, often five or six, until I could stop shivering. As I got warm, I would drift off into the soundest few hours of sleep I could get.

Going to the spray table was a one to two hour ordeal. Everything about it was uncomfortable for me, starting with the transfer from my bed to the stainless steel table on wheels. Just lying on it was painful. Now that the left half of my back was merely ribs and an eighth of an inch of skin, I didn't have any muscle or soft-tissue padding there. The nurses used the sheets under me to do the transfer, so once it was done the sheet had to be taken out. They would roll me one direction, stuffing that half of the sheet underneath me, then roll me the other way so all the sheet could be removed. This was followed by moving me in all directions to remove my bandages. Then came the bathing part where they washed me, scrubbed me, and cared for my wounds. The spray rooms were equipped with retractable hoses and sprayers, which reminded me of what an industrial dishwashing sprayer looks like. To this day I cannot understand why they had to use cold water to do their work on me. I would freeze, lying their naked, shivering and begging them to make the water warmer. My teeth often chattered so hard I felt like I was going to start chipping them. The excuse was always that it had something to do with the old plumbing. Once in a while I was fortunate enough to get some warmer water. The wound care involved removing staples and the covering materials from the grafts and donor sites as they became loose and slowly came off. The donor sites stung so badly from the water, cleaning or any pressure. I finally resorted to trying to negotiate, I was so desperate to reduce the pain wherever I could. The nurses were very understanding but definitely followed their orders and did the job they had to do. They did accomodate my wishes whenever they could. Once the torture was complete, everything was bandaged up and we headed back to my room, where I was transferred again into my clean bed. It was a long, tiresome procedure for everyone involved.

My room in the burn unit at Metro had some memorable aspects. I did have a window, out of which I could see some sunlight, buildings, and most interestingly, the takeoff and landing of the rescue helicopter. The room had a little vestibule on the outside of my room where all visitors had to get dressed up and wash their hands prior to coming into my room. While I was on the critical side of the burn unit, all the people that came into my room had to wear hair covering, masks, gloves, and gowns. The protective clothing was uncomfortable and hot for everyone, but necessary to protect my open wounds from infection. Other aspects of my room included a painting of some battle with the Texas flag prominently in the center. This painting was just below my TV. I never understood why that particular one was chosen, but I interpreted it as signifying the battle for life that many patients in that bed had to fight. I had a small TV with about six channels and without my beloved ESPN, I was very sad. I had so much time to watch TV, it would have been nice to have my favorite channel. Michelle had wallpapered the remaining spaces with cards from all well-wishers, and with pictures of her, the kids, and our new house in Pennsylvania. I also had some of the kids' artwork on the walls. These paintings were so nice to see, but were also a sad reminder of the fact that I wasn't there to be with them, and I hadn't seen them for such a long time.

Journal Entry - 5/21/00

Yesterday and today were pretty blah days for you both emotionally and physically. Your stomach still doesn't feel so hot and you've been pretty bummed I think (and so you said). I felt bad today because it was the first day that someone was not with you the entire day. You were expecting us in the AM and when I called in at 10:45 you were resting, so we decided to have an early lunch then come in. When we got there you were in the dreaded cardiac chair (the torture chair as you called it to Leron).

Anyway, I felt bad for you today and all of this that you are having to go through and deal with. I know everything right now is or seems like a big struggle and that has to be hard to handle especially since you were so healthy and strong right before this. I encouraged you to do a little each day and build on each as you can to reach that ultimate goal of OUT OF HERE!! You did some PT with me today-even leg lifts that you said were "too hard," and I was proud of you for trying a little. At least it is a place to start. I told you and you tried to drink some Boost for me too. I love you baby and I don't want to push you too hard but I don't want you to be in that bed any longer than you have to be either, so I'll help you as I can. Tomorrow is Monday and they will look at your grafts again, so I want to be there to talk with the Dr.'s. I told you I would be there, which you seemed glad about. So I am going to hit the sack now and get six hours before a.m. I love you sweetheart, and I can't wait until it's not annoying to you for me to touch you. I'm not taking it personally, but it is hard, I do miss you immensely!!! XOXOXO to you babe. See you in the morning. M-

Taylor and Chase were also victims of this illness. At ages four and two, I'm sure they had no idea what was really going on. It was obvious to them that life as they knew it had been turned upside-down. Mommy was very busy and away from the house for long periods of time, and daddy was suddenly taken completely from their lives. There was still talk about him and how he was sick, but it had to be hard for them to understand the severity of daddy's illness. They did get to spend large amounts of time with grandparents, other family, and friends which was nice but certainly couldn't replace the mommy and daddy-time. Michelle and social workers had discussed when the best time would be for the boys to visit. The advice had been to wait until I could at least communicate with them and looked similar to the state they were used to seeing me in. The social workers and child-life specialists had done such a great job helping Michelle and the rest of the family through this. Their help in preparing the boys for seeing me was invaluable. They even took the time to put together a doll that had a tube in its nose, an IV in its arm, an airplane splint on the other arm and wrapped in ace bandages in order to give them an idea of what I looked like before they saw me. I remember being extremely nervous prior to them coming. I wasn't sure how they would react to me in my sickly state. Their visit was a big deal for everybody on the unit. Everyone there had spent so much time with Michelle and me, they were anxious to meet the boys and witness our reunion.

The visit went pretty well, as well as anyone could have expected them to do under such difficult circumstances. The boys were given lots of gifts and treats in an attempt to make it a very positive experience. I found it very difficult to talk with them, I kept trying to engage them but it was obvious they were still uncomfortable with the way I looked and with the entire setting. Taylor is naturally quiet, so even though he seemed to sense that things were going well with me, his responses to my questions were short. He had a very hard time looking at me or making eye contact. Chase is much more open but was obviously overwhelmed with seeing me so thin, bandaged, and weak that he didn't say much either. I felt so bad for them, putting them through such a difficult experience, but it did allow them to start making the necessary adjustments to better understand our situation. Every visit that followed got better and better for them, as they grew more accustomed to seeing me at the hospital. I always had mixed feelings when they visited, I was so glad to be seeing them but so saddened by our separation and the trauma my illness was causing them. Seeing them in person brought out extreme emotions in me, appropriately for such an ordeal. What did they do to deserve such a wrench in their lives, to have a dad that looked strange and sick? I worried about how they would respond. Would they be scarred long-term from going through this? It certainly changes your perspective on pain, physical and emotional. I, as most parents, would much rather hurt than to have my children suffer. Unfortunately, kids must endure stressful situations all of the time. Try as we might, parents cannot completely shield their kids from stress.

Journal Entry - 5/23/00

Let me back up again and tell you about yesterday. As I write this, I am sitting in the motor home with the boys trying to nap and the packers are here inside the house making great headway. Chase is driving me crazy at the moment, not lying still and not listening at all. My patience is very thin as well from lack of sleep, so that does not help. Your parents have left to come in and see you, and then I will come in at dinnertime for the evening. I must admit I am pretty spent today and will be glad to relax more tomorrow. Chase is so sad at this moment - won't lay down so I have sat here right next to him. Finally I rubbed his back and sang songs, so now he is out. Now Taylor to deal with. Funny how he has to go potty again - just went - too bad. The potty out here is pretty exciting you know. It is lightly raining outside now - kind of peaceful , especially if they were both sleeping. I just got my 10 minute power nap and feel a little better. Anyway about yesterday, they looked at your skin grafts again and Dr. Frat said 85 to 90 percent now because a few small spots have come loose. He is still really pleased with how things look and is also very pleased with your physical condition (strength). I know you feel very weak, but it'll all come back with a little persistence each day. I wish I could make all this easier for you, but unfortunately I can't. They had you leaning over the side of your bed today for your dressing change and Tami was there to make sure you were in good position and could handle it all. She said you had to work hard but you handled it wonderfully. They wrapped you in ace bandages this time and took all your drains out, so each new day a little more progress!

You are also less nauseated too. Then in the afternoon, the boys came in to see you for the first time. They each picked out a balloon for you from the grocery store. Chase chose Burt and Taylor chose Mickey Mouse. Your mom and I got you one that said "B-well" with a bee on it. They were excited to bring them to you. Jill, the child-life specialist, met with us beforehand to explain things to the boys. She showed them the picture book of your room and the things in it, and a doll with his arm wrapped in ace bandages like you. You obviously were aware of the whole visit so I don't need to write details. I think they loved the bears you gave them and the megablocks bus has been a real hit - even so much they're having great difficulty sharing at times. They also loved the popsicles and so did you! I was thrilled to see you eat a whole twin pop by yourself and enjoy it! As I said, a little progress each day is wonderful (in any area)! I think they both thought you looked different - Taylor had a hard time looking at you, but did talk with you and neither of them were scared. Chase today said he wanted his "different" daddy again. I tried to explain he only has one daddy and you're in the hospital and you will come home again soon - when you're better. I wish they could understand better.

I spent the morning with you and into the afternoon - they did your dressing change in your room at 1:30, and I spoke with Dr. Frat afterwards. His big concern is the reconstruction of your armpit. He needs to consult with Dr. Goldstein about what needs to be done and at which hospital. I did speak with Dr. Goldstein on the phone last night as he was leaving Metro from visiting you and he said he was going to call Dr. Fratianne and arrange a time to see you during a dressing change.

So, today I have not been able to come in and see you because of the movers being here. I miss you so much punkin! Well, a short nap for Chase because one of the movers came out with a question for me. Oh my, a rainy day in a confined area is not good. I was just on the phone with Ethan and the boys were acting up a lot, which I've been told has been an ongoing problem. So they both are now in time-out. Joy! It's only three o'clock and I hope the movers get done soon. I wish I could take the boys somewhere and it would be easier, but I really can't leave with the movers here - especially since they may have questions about what stays versus goes.

So, I'll be patient! Can't wait to see you tonight! I sure hope you're having a good day. Your nurse Chris said you stood up from bed during your dressing change today - WOW! Impressive babe. So glad to hear of your strength and progress each day! You can do it sweetie. I love you. M-

My recovery continued through the end of May, with each day bringing new challenges and small strides towards recovery. The therapists were doing lots of work on both of my legs and on my left shoulder. One of the devices that was used to increase my strength and ability to sit was something called a cardiac chair. This is a special chair which starts laid out flat, and then can be slowly adjusted, cranking the back up slowly to the desired height. I'm not exaggerating at all when I say that I hated that chair. I hated it with a passion. I referred to it as my torture chair. Sitting in that chair was almost as awful as getting scrubbed on the spray table. Sitting in the chair was not only a positive step toward increasing my strength, but also served as a negative focus for all the anger built up through my illness. I guess this was better than taking my anger out on other people. I remember very vividly one afternoon, the nurses demanded I sit in the chair, and my friend Leron happened to come for a visit. Leron was also a pediatric resident and was a great support to Michelle and me throughout the entire illness. He had taken time from his busy schedule to travel across town to see me, and I always tried to put on my best game-face whenever I had company. I felt so bad as I sat there in such agony, with sweat pouring down my face as I tried to maintain a conversation with him. I was nauseated, hurting all over and feeling terrible. I know he felt bad too, seeing me sit there in such discomfort. It is still amazing to look back at how weak I really was, to be so uncomfortable just from sitting up. From that point on I always did my best to make sure that I wasn't in the chair if any visitors were coming.

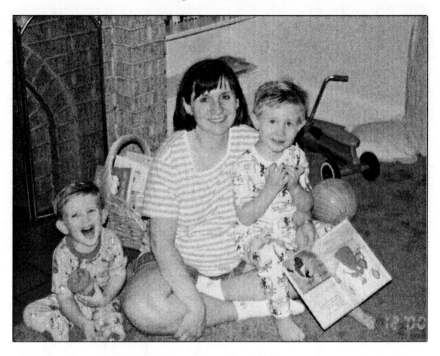

Michelle, Taylor and Chase reading
some books together in our apartment.

I was fortunate to have so many visitors. I know many people don't have that luxury when they are in the hospital. While I was at University Hospitals ICU during the first part of my illness, friends, family and colleagues from Rainbow were a constant presence there, at times taking over the waiting room. After my most critical first week when she was there constantly, Michelle came to see me every day. Sometimes she stayed for the whole day, sometimes for a couple hours depending on what was going on at home. My parents, who had arrived on Easter Sunday, had stayed for six weeks, with my mom actually staying for the entire summer. Without her there as summer progressed, Michelle would have only been able to come see me sporadically when she could find someone to watch the kids. In addition to all the aforementioned folks, we had visits from the Roth's, Cimbala's, Corrado's and Larry Connor during this time. It was so great for all these folks to come, and all of them helped out so much in one way or another. Everybody rotated taking turns watching the children and visiting me. As if the stress of my illness wasn't enough, we also had to worry about moving, we had sold our house in Cleveland Heights prior to my illness. Michelle had to take time to look for a temporary place to live until I was strong enough to finish my residency and move to Pennsylvania. After looking with no success, an incredible opportunity opened up for a small two-bedroom apartment only about 10 minutes from Metro hospital. A former Rainbow resident was living with his wife in a two-family house in Lakewood, and were only living in half of the house. After hearing of our predicament, they offered to let us stay there, and we gladly accepted. The majority of our belongings were packed up and moved to our new house in Pennsylvania, only the bare essentials were moved to the apartment. Mattresses were laid on the floor, the furniture consisted of lawn chairs, privacy was at a minimum, but it served our purpose well. We will always be grateful to the Vogelgesang's for helping us out in our difficult situation. We gave Michelle's parents power of attorney so that they could close on our house in Pennsylvania, and Michelle's dad took over our finances. It was truly a team effort to get us through, and we will always be indebted to everyone who helped us out. I felt so helpless lying there in the hospital bed while everyone else was doing the jobs that I normally did. Sometimes you feel like you cannot say thank you enough.

Meanwhile, my recovery continued to go as well as expected. It took about two weeks for the extreme burning pain from my donor sites to begin easing up. That helped tremendously, allowing me to put forth more effort to increase my strength and mobility.

Chapter 7

Step-Down Unit

A bout two weeks after my grafting surgery, I was moved to the step-down section of the burn unit. This area was adjacent to the "critical" side of the unit and was for patients who didn't require one-on-one nursing, ventilators, central lines and constant monitoring. Everything was more relaxed on this side, helping make everyone feel more comfortable. It was nice that visitors were no longer required to wear gowns, masks, and gloves when they entered my room. They were still required to wash their hands.

In terms of my medical care, the big question remained as to what to do with my armpit and the large concave defect under my left shoulder blade. Several different options had been discussed, but none of them seemed very reasonable to me. Because it was such a large defect, and because of the constant motion of the shoulder blade, traditional skin grafting was unlikely to succeed. Dr. Kaufman, a plastic surgeon at Metro, was consulted to help. There was no obvious solution to the dilemma, so more and more opinions were sought, trying to develop the best plan to cover this area. Dr. Kaufman even talked to several colleagues across the country, trying to talk to someone who had been in a similar situation or had a fresh idea. One frequently discussed option included taking the latissimus muscle, the muscle which makes up the back of your armpit, from my good, right side and surgically moving it over to the left covering the defect. A traditional skin graft placed overtop would then have something more structured to adhere to. I was adamantly against this option because I felt it was most important to have at least one strong shoulder, and I didn't want them weakening my right side just to patch my left. Without knowing what function I would have on the left, I really wanted to leave the right untouched. Another option was to actually reduce the size of the defect by cutting off the bottom section of my left shoulder blade, which was serving no purpose since all the muscle attachments on the bottom half had already been removed during the initial surgeries. With the bottom of my shoulder blade gone, a smaller defect would be left, one which the surgeons felt a full-thickness graft from my left forearm could adequately cover. A full-thickness graft takes the skin and all the soft tissue from an area. Because it is thicker then a skin graft, it requires a blood supply to be transferred with it, enabling its survival in its new location. Regular skin grafts actually grow their own microscopic blood vessels to keep the tissues alive after transfer. The extra thickness of this type of graft would make it more durable and more likely to survive in an area like the armpit. The surgery would involve removing a large patch from the underside of my left forearm, with parts of the radial artery and vein included, and transferring it to the defect area. Then, Dr. Kaufman would "plumb in" the artery and vein to a large artery and vein in my armpit. A regular skin graft would then be taken from remaining good skin to cover the exposed muscle on my forearm. After lots of discussion and planning, this second option became everyone's choice. I was willing to lose a little bit cosmetically on my left arm to keep my right shoulder strong.

The day of my surgery came on May 31st, Michelle and my eighth wedding anniversary. Since the surgery was going to involve three different surgeons, we couldn't be fussy on the date. We had to do it when all the surgeons were available at the same time. I was nervous as I always was prior to surgery, but tried to keep reminding myself that every hurdle was one step closer to the prize. That didn't seem to slow the 500-pound butterflies crisscrossing through my stomach.

The surgery itself was a multi-step process, a real team effort. Drs. Kaufman and Fratianne, as well as Dr. Lacey, an orthopedic surgeon, all had roles. First, the bottom half of my shoulder blade needed to be removed by Dr. Lacey. Removing bone is a pretty gruesome process where special saws take off the necessary parts. Dr. Kaufman would then harvest the full-thickness graft from my forearm. This part was very meticulous as all the vessels attached to the graft were dissected out, the remaining vessels tied off and the graft vessels resewn at their new location. This meant a reimplantation in my armpit area of the full-thickness graft with surrounding skin grafts. This would be done in conjunction with Dr. Fratianne. Finally, a new skin graft would be taken to cover the newly-created defect on my forearm. Due to operating room scheduling, they hadn't been able to start the surgery till late afternoon. We knew the surgery would be lengthy, and indeed it was, going well into the night. Things weren't finished until around 12:30 AM, and I wasn't out of recovery until 2:30 AM. This meant a long night for both the surgeons and for my family anxiously awaiting to hear how the surgery went. All this effort was worthwhile though. The surgery went well, without complications. The true measure of success from this challenging surgery wouldn't be known for a few days, while we waited to see how things healed. Everyone was exhausted and happy to be through the long ordeal. This wouldn't be my last surgery. The flap would need to heal and solidify before the final grafting on the back part of my shoulder could be attached to it. The likelihood of success was too small if it was done all at once. I wasn't excited to think about going to surgery again, but it was nice knowing that the most complex and difficult operation was over.

In talking with Dr. Fratianne years later, it was amazing and almost scary to think about how truly difficult the reconstruction of my armpit was. He talked about how they had a basic plan for the surgery going in, but the results were very dynamic in that during each step of the surgery they had to stop and try to gauge what the particular actions would mean for my healing and ultimately my long-term function and protection. In this type of surgery, the decades of experience from all those involved couldn't have been more useful and important as they attempted something they had never done before. They knew they were treading in unchartered waters and any mistakes would be catastrophic for me. I was already sacrificing some of my forearm, if the surgery didn't work, what would be next?

When they were finished, I was stable, quickly extubated and brought back to my room on the step-down unit. I saw Michelle and my mom briefly before they headed home to get some sleep. I was pretty groggy but didn't feel too badly considering all the cutting and manipulating I had been through.

Journal Entry - 5/31/00

Happy Anniversary Sweetheart! So sorry that on this day you have to be here and also in surgery. I am sitting in your room with George Winston playing and thinking of you. Just a moment as I pause to say another prayer. They just called up from the OR and just began the actual surgery (4:18 pm). I left you at 3:00 from the surgery holding-area as they wheeled you in. You had a tear in your eye after saying goodbye and I love you. I just cried on my way back up to the burn unit. Oh

- *this is so hard to see you have to endure so much! In all the past surgeries we had **so** many people aware and praying and I feel like not everyone knows about this today. But I also know that the most important person - the Lord - knows and that is what matters. "God will take care of you, through every day, ore' all the way, He will take care of you, God will take care of you."*

3 Peter 5:7 "Cast all your cares upon Him, for He careth for you."

Laurel just called to check in and see how things are going, so I talked with her a bit. 6:00 - the receptionist just gave me a report from the OR that everything is going well and as planned! Thank the Lord!! We will continue to pray for you baby! I know that it will all be okay - God has brought you so far already! I know that this surgery is harder on you emotionally than any of the others because you are much more aware, but I hope it won't be any more stressful on your body because you are stronger than you have been in the past. It sounds like I will stay here at the hospital for the whole surgery - I just can't bear the thought of leaving at all. I think the plan is now for your parents to bring in the kids for a bit and then your mom to stay maybe. I don't know, we'll see. Maybe it is selfish of me to feel like this, but...

Your dinner just came and of course, it looks like a dinner you would actually like: fried chicken, potatoes and gravy, peaches, a roll, salad with Ranch dressing, and you are not able to eat it. I ate the salad and a bite of the other things - you are right - nothing tastes that great. We'll need to bring in better food for you after you are feeling up to it. Maybe then you'll feel more up to eating too. It is now 6:50 - time goes by so slowly when you have to patiently wait.

Ahh! Big sigh - 6:55. Dr. Kaufman just came to see me - they are taking a brief break - the flap is off, totally dissected and they are giving it time to perfuse before putting it in. The armpit area is all cleaned up and ready to go too. So they will continue. He said he plans to hook up the vessels into those in your upper arm and thinks that will work out well. He said it is hard to see all the way up into your armpit, he will have to use the magnifying glasses since he can't use the microscope. So I will say another prayer now.

Your Dad just called - they were all ready to come in when the severe storm sirens began sounding and it started pouring, so they are waiting it out. And it sounds like they are getting an 80% burn victim in, so my adrenalin is going up at the moment. No - I just heard the patient is only an 8% burn - that's good. But still worried about the kids being scared without me there and worried about you too. All are in good hands though, I remind myself. Sounds nasty outside - hope it moves through quickly so nothing happens here. To add to all this, the little boy next door to you here is all worked up as they try to take off his dressings.

Okay, things are better now. The boys and your parents came in for a visit, so that was nice. Taylor was sad leaving though, didn't understand why both me and Grandma had to stay. I didn't get in as much time with them as I would have liked though because my parents called and so did Dr. Goldstein for an update. The boys and your Dad left about 9:30 so your Mom and I are here. Lisa, the nurse, asked if you were coming back and I said no, I haven't heard anything since a little before 7:00 and would just like to know that they are still working and that things are going well. So she said she would call down and try to find out for us. I told her that would be very sweet. So........it is 9:50 and they said all is going well and blood flow is good, but still need to graft your forearm, so it'll be another one and a half hours until you are done. Sigh. Long day for all. We'll say another prayer now, and write more later. Your Mom and I are waiting in the "fish room." All my love being sent your way sweetie.

Well, 10:15 now - Lisa came back and said the OR called and your graft is on and they are just sewing you up. All is still going well and they are planning on extubating you in the PACU and then after recovering there they'll bring you up to your room. So, I do pray that all that will go smoothly for you. Just another Praise the Lord that it has gone well and almost over for you again. We'll hate to leave you again tonight. You were so "you" before going in, I just don't know what to expect this time, especially if you will already be extubated. At any rate, we will be here for a while with you. I hope your Mom doesn't mind being here late - she said not.

We just figured out that this is your 6ᵗʰ surgery since this all began, including the original lipoma operation. Wow - I hadn't really thought about it specifically. 12:20 am. Still no word from the Doc's and PACU hasn't called up yet - I'm a bit worried, but shouldn't be since they said it would be a few hours until you'd be up. So hard to wait!!! I just wish Dr. Kaufman would come talk to us. Guess what? Janie, your nurse just came in and said he'd be right up - what timing! Can't wait to hear. Your Mom and I are sitting here in the "fish room" with blankets on (Janie got for us) since it is so cold in here and we have shorts on.

They said you are in recovery right now too (12:30). Janie is your nurse tonight, so I am glad - my comfort level leaving you will be better having someone who has been with you a lot here after a big day like this. But I will still not rest easy, I'm sure.

Dr. Kaufman just came and said he thought everything went really well. He did say you lost more blood than normal because he had to stop blood flow in two areas of that left arm and didn't want it to get stagnant and cause a thrombosis, so he gave you Heparin to eliminate that possibility before you lost a bit more. He said he checked your crit afterwards and it was at 27 - not much different than when you went in. But he said it would be likely that your fluids would shift during the night and they would maybe have to give you a few units of blood. (Lost about 350 cc of blood). The flap seems to be working well. He said you had big easy vessels to sew, and used the two biggest (I've forgotten their names already) in your upper arm to join the flap to. The flap itself has no dressing on it because Dr. Kaufman doesn't want it restricted in any way, so we'll get to see it. They did take off your biobrane on the back of your thighs and you bled some but looks okay I guess. And they did have the corpack feeding tube put back in but of course we'll have to have an x-ray to check its placement. And you were extubated right away with no problems - I am happy for you babe! I called Dr. Goldstein at 1:05 am, because he told me to, no matter what the time, but I felt wrong doing it. He had called earlier tonight for an update and said to call him. He is planning to come in the morning to see you if you are not asleep. I'm debating on whether to stay here tonight or go home - not sure what they'll allow me to do, we'll see. Janie went down to get you (1:45 am), so anxious to see you. Will write more tomorrow, because I might be too tired tonight to write again after I see you. M-

Psalm 100 - *too much to write but it is a psalm for giving thanks. It's short to read though. (We have included it here for you)*

"Shout for joy to the Lord, all the earth. Worship the Lord with gladness; come before him with joyful songs. Know that the Lord is God. It is he who made us, and we are his; we are his people, the sheep of his pasture. Enter His gates with thanksgiving and His courts with praise; give thanks to Him and praise His name. For the Lord is good and His love endures forever; His faithfulness continues through all generations."

6/1/00

8:00 am. I am back here this morning to see you after only two hours of sleep. I tried to call this morning to get an update on you at 6:40, but no one answered so I still don't have any info since I left you about 3:30 am. The doctors are rounding on you now, so I can't go in yet, I would like to have some info as soon as possible. Don't see a receptionist or nurse near the front here at all to even ask - frustrating. But I guess everyone or almost everyone is busy.

Its now to 12:20 and I am at home after only seeing you a bit this morning. Dr. Fratianne reamed me out in the good way for being there so soon this morning and told me to give you a kiss and go home. He said I needed to worry about me and baby and let them worry about you since you are doing fine. Nice for people to be con-

cerned I guess. Anyway, I did not go home immediately and I'm glad I didn't as I was there when Dr. Kaufman came in and said he thought everything looked good. Dr. Goldstein came after and agreed. They are dopplering the flap every hour for good blood flow and so far so good. They are giving you blood since your crit was at 23. They ultrasounded your legs for clots and that turned out normal too. So I stayed for a bit after that and then they wanted to mess with your tubing and take you in for a dressing change at 10:30, you told me to go home at that point and I said that I would let you rest afterwards. You're in a lot of pain and you're going to get more morphine during your dressing change. I called a 12:30 then and Amy, your nurse, said that she thought you did pretty well during your dressing change and you are resting. So maybe come in the see you around 3:00 so that you can get in a good nap.

I came in myself, got here at 4:15 and we visited until 7:30 and I left you to take a nap while I was going to get something to eat. Unfortunately I had to come right back because the cafeteria is closed. I've forgot. Oh well, I'll eat at home, no biggie. As I look at you while you are

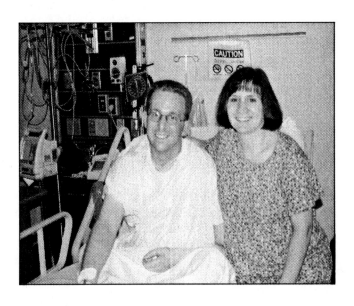

Craig in his hospital bed with Michelle after his full-thickness graft surgery.

sleeping I can't help but think "thank you Lord!" For who you are and what he has done for you to allow you to still be here with me! I love you so much sweetie and just can't wait to show you - just want to hold you *and love you. I know I keep telling you this, but it is true. They say you don't know what you've got until its gone - while I did know what I had prior to this time, I am ever so thankful that you are not gone! You're awake now - half-hour later, because the nurse needed to come in to do vitals. M-*

Communication is such an integral part of providing quality health care. Poor communication, as is often the case, leads to misunderstanding. When physicians and families don't communicate accurately with one another, misconceptions frequently occur. That is why it is optimal to be present and speak to physicians in person, rather than speaking with physicians by phone. Inflections given by physicians when they speak, as well as the ability for doctors to fully bring the family up to speed and assess their understanding work so much better in person. Especially during times of stress, that face-to-face meeting with the patient's physician is so crucial to understanding each individual condition. Michelle tried so hard to be around when she could speak with the doctors, and after I was awake I tried to talk with them as much as possible. I was so fortunate to have such good people taking care of me. This has led to continued relationships even years after my illness has resolved.

One thing that always got to me while I was awake in the hospital was being shaved. It is a very humbling experience to have someone drag a razor across your face, especially the ones they used in the hospital. I didn't get shaved everyday, so when I did it was quite a production. The first time I was awake and really with it, I couldn't believe how much it hurt. Being shaved with these cheap white razors with one so-called blade felt as if my whiskers were being pulled out one at a time instead of shaved off. I was a little surprised these razors were legal on the very strict burn unit, my face was left with a bunch of little nicks. I finally asked Michelle to pick up some real razors at the store and bring them in for the nurses to use.

During this stage of my recovery, one of the goals we put forward was to be able to leave the hospital for an evening to attend my Rainbow Senior Resident dinner. This dinner is an informal occasion to get all the senior residents together one last time before going on to their new jobs or fellowships. Held in a local restaurant, the event consisted of a sit-down dinner and culminated in a "roasting" of the seniors by the intern, first year, class of residents. Even while knowing such a long night would be a struggle, I really wanted to go. I wanted to see some people one last time, and to prove to myself and everyone else that I could do it. With my goal-oriented personality, it was beneficial for me to have specific things to strive for and work towards. We talked about the plans with everyone at Metro and they were all very supportive of the idea. Rainbow and Metro are semi-competitive institutions, so there were always somewhat funny feelings from the Metro staff towards Rainbow visitors coming to see me, or any mention of Rainbow in their presence. Despite this, my senior night became a goal for everyone on the team.

Before going to my senior dinner, I really wanted to get the feeding tube out of my nose. Not only was it irritating, but it wouldn't look good going outside the hospital. Every time a nurse flushed the darned thing it would make me nauseous. Still, I was not feeling that great, so I wasn't eating much. The nutritionists and dietitians seemed so intent on getting me to eat lots of calories. I felt as if my appetite would increase with the feeding tube gone. Along with my regular meals, they had been trying to get me to drink Boost shakes for some extra calories. They didn't taste all that bad, but the most I could do in a day along with my regular meals was to drink one or two. I kept asking what it would take to get the feeding tube out of my nose. Finally they decided that if I could drink ten Boosts in one day, they would remove the feeding tube. I think they truly thought I couldn't do it, but they underestimated how determined I was to get that hose out of my nose. I didn't eat anything else that day, I just drank Boosts until I thought I might croak. Nevertheless, I reached their goal and late in the evening finished my tenth Boost. And as promised, they removed the tube. As nauseous as that tube made me feel while it was in place, it was no surprise that when they removed it I vomited several Boosts with it. I didn't care though, at last it was gone. The next day, the nutritionists came in and said that they had misunderstood, I didn't need to drink that many Boosts in one day. That was good because I'm not sure I could handle another day like that one. I promised to do my best to put as many calories in me as possible.

Journal Entry - 6/4/00

Sorry for not writing for several days again, just haven't had the time. A synopsis of the past few days is: Friday - your mom and dad came in to see you after lunch, I didn't come in until after dinner. It was a long day not seeing you until the evening, but it was a good long evening together. I stayed until midnight. Saturday - your mom and dad came in to see you immediately after your dressing change in the morning and then I met them here to take your dad to the airport. The boys enjoyed seeing all the planes and activity and we had a Burger King lunch there as well. My parents arrived while we were gone, had lunch, and then came in to see you. I met them here on the way home from the airport while your mom took two napping boys home. We didn't stay very long as you were really in need of a nap. Then my parents, the boys and I came in around 7 PM. Taylor and Chase gave you the cards they drew. You sat in a chair the whole time - and as soon as they left you threw up, had your armpit dressing change and were whipped, so I went home about 10:15. Now it is Sunday and your mom went to church, my parents are with the boys and I came in here for 45 minutes before they took you for a dressing change. I just spoke with Dr. Yowler and he feels that the redness may just be a yeast infection, but if it is some other superficial skin infection, that change last night of putting you back on Vancomycin should help. Otherwise your flap and grafts look real good. He said there are two patchy areas as big as his hand that will need to be grafted again, but the question is when. He wants to do it sooner than later but wants to consult Dr. Frat before any decisions. He said this coming week needs to be intense physical therapy, though the question is where? Here at the burn unit, the rehab unit at Metro, or elsewhere. So, some questions need to be decided upon and we'll go from there. I talked with him also about your nausea and throwing up patterns and he said he would check the drugs you are on to see, but he is still not too worried about you much (and neither am I - I know you will eat when you feel up to it, like you were prior to surgery). Everyone else seems more upset with you, wanting you to eat. I kind of got the cold shoulder from a nurse today I felt - not sure why. Maybe they're sick of me here , I don't know. Oh well, it's a plus being here so much - I think. I hope you think so.

Oh, back to Dr. Yowler's time-line thoughts. He said we will try to plan your grafting surgery for June 14th so you can go to your senior dinner. He recommended doing the surgery the week of the 12th, I mentioned the dinner and he said doing Wednesday vs. Monday is not much difference, so no problem. Then here for five days following and then PT either at a rehab hospital or at home depending on your needs. So maybe two to three weeks more for sure, then??? He also said another scenario would be to do physical therapy for two weeks, then do your surgery, but if it were up to him, he'd like to do the surgery sooner. I knew you'd be happier with that option! Well, I'm going to see if you're done, because I have to go for the big chicken dinner my mom is making for all, then my parents will be in this afternoon before they go home to Pennsylvania. M-

The nurses and staff were great as we prepared for the dinner. They arranged for my mom to go out and get a corsage so I could give it to Michelle as we left for the dinner. I felt a little silly, we weren't going to the prom, but it was easier to go along than resist all my nurse's wishes. They even made the effort to find a shiny new wheelchair from another floor, as they didn't want me going out looking shabby. I was concerned about having the stamina to sit up for such a long period of time, but I was determined to make it.

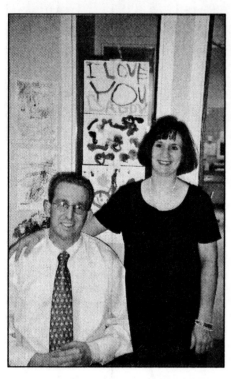

Craig and Michelle ready to go to his Senior Dinner. Notice the kid's artwork behind.

Finally, the big night arrived in mid-June. I decided that I wanted to wear a tie, even though nobody would have worried if I wasn't wearing one. Michelle brought in some dress clothes for me. What a task it was just to get them on. Here I was, having not worn any real clothes for months, trying to get into pants, a button-down shirt, and a tie. Fortunately, we had given ourselves lots of time to get dressed. Between my significant weight loss and my bandages everywhere, the clothes didn't fit like they had before, but we finally got them on. My resident friends John and Leron agreed to come and pick us up, then return us to the hospital after the dinner. I had an intense feeling of excitement, getting wheeled off the burn unit in civilian clothes. You would have thought I had just gotten out of prison.

Many parts of the night were memorable. I remember the car ride to the restaurant very well. The open wound in my back was so sensitive, every bump in the road felt like a new knife, stabbing into my back. Since Cleveland usually gets a lot of snow in the winter, frequent snow plow activity created greater than its fair share of potholes and rough roads. I just had to grin and bear it, the rough ride could not be avoided if I wanted to get to my dinner.

Arriving after the tortuous ride, we soon found out first-hand how hard getting around in a wheelchair was. The restaurant was a small Italian place in a very old building, located in an older area of Cleveland Heights, known as Coventry. Coventry is a couple of blocks of quaint, older buildings with many shops, restaurants and theaters. At our particular restaurant, the only wheelchair access was a ramp in the back that ran right next to several garbage dumpsters that smelled as if they hadn't been emptied in weeks. What a cruel joke, getting out of the hospital for the first time and my first smell of freedom was garbage.

We were able to make our way in, but getting through the walk-ways and between the tables was also a real challenge as everything was very cramped and narrow. Once we finally made our way in, I got the impression that everyone was glad I was there, but it was obvious that it was hard for everyone to know what to say to Michelle and me. What emotions we must have brought out in my classmates, to see one of their own in such a bad state. Once a strapping young doctor, I'd been pushed to the brink of death, now thin, weak, and confined to a wheelchair. Who better than this group of physicians to know the hell we had been through and still had ahead of us in my rehabilitation. We were so thankful for everyone's support, it was hard to imagine a more generous and helpful group than the administration, staff, and residents at Rainbow.

My meal was a large steak dinner that I barely put a dent in, my appetite was far from it's usual. After dinner the "roasting" began, as the interns had put together a program of popular music songs to describe each senior. As they played them, all the seniors tried to guess which senior each group of songs symbolized. Most of the music collections were hilarious, and it made for a very pleasant and entertaining evening. When you work so many hours with people, you get to know them very well, their qualities and quirks. I'm not sure where they found it, but for my songs the interns played the theme from "Welcome Back, Kotter," followed by the "Rocky" theme song. It was a moving time for all of us, followed by many hugs and a few tears from everyone. Afterwards, Michelle and I were presented a large check from money that had been collected for us by everyone at Rainbow. We were overwhelmed. The money was so helpful as we tried to stay afloat, paying on two residences with only my minimal disability-income. As happened throughout my entire illness, God provided and everyone's generosity abounded for us.

As the evening wrapped up, we headed back to the hospital, ending my brief furlough. We can't remember how late we got back, but we did stay out late enough to get all the nurses into an uproar. Everyone was so worried about me not being able to handle the stress and energy required, but I did just fine. I was thoroughly exhausted and sore when I got back. I remember not wanting to take the time to get undressed, but without a choice in this matter, I was quickly helped out of my clothes and into bed. I slept very well, and I think everyone else felt better once I was back in the hospital, safe and sound.

Journal Entry - July 2000

Dear Craig and Michelle:

You two are so inspiring- you are the reason I get up in the morning! Your strength and courage fulfill me - I feed off of it!! Craig - your example of faith will always be with me to inspire me when I am in need. Michelle - your devotion and dedication to your husband and family makes me strive to be a better person. God bless you and your family. Love, Tami K. (The physical "terrorist")

You know I just couldn't write one thing. I had to add the poem that Shannon and I wrote (Shannon wrote the good part!)

Roses are red, Violets are blue, You are healed, Now goodbye to you!!

Truly, best wishes. Words cannot convey what strength you have given me. TK

As my medical condition continued to improve, the focus of my care was starting to shift towards rehabilitation. The team decided the best move would be to transfer me to a rehabilitation floor within the same hospital. I could still travel down to the burn unit for dressing changes, but moving would give me the opportunity for several hours of occupational and physical therapy everyday. The rehab floor had all the necessary tools and therapists who could devote more time to me. It is a well-known fact of human nature that most people are against change, and I was very apprehensive about leaving the burn unit. I was used to the routines, the nurses and staff, and all my doctors on the burn unit. I didn't see why I couldn't just go to the rehab floor for the rehab and stay the rest of the time in my comfort zone. I'm sure money and the expense of each hospital day in the two locales played a large role in the decision-making. Despite trying to negotiate, I was moved off the burn unit to the rehab floor for what was projected to be a two-to-three week stay.

Chapter 8

Rehabilitation

I don't recall having a real bad attitude going into my transfer, but it didn't take long to figure out that I really disliked the conditions on the rehab floor. I don't want to spend a lot of time bad-mouthing anyone, but all the things that made the burn unit run so well were missing on the rehab unit. In my opinion, it was dirty, smelly, overcrowded and understaffed. The most dramatic example was the obvious feces that were smeared on the wall of my bathroom when I moved in. I always felt like I was pulling teeth to get any help there. The people that worked there were very nice, just stretched too thin to get all the work done. I was very motivated to progress through my rehabilitation as fast as possible. I knew I was going home as soon as I was strong enough.

Job 23:10 "He knoweth the way that I take: when He has tried me, I shall come forth as gold."

The days on the rehab floor were tough with between two and three hours of therapy each day. Jen, my occupational therapist, and Adrian, my physical therapist, were both great and pushed me very hard. My therapy sessions were split so that

I did have some rest periods in between, which was necessary to keep me going through the painful and tiring rehab work. After dinner time, I would have my shower, sitting as I couldn't stand long enough, in the rehab unit, then get wheeled to the burn unit for my daily dressing change. I was so weak by this time of day my nurse had to do all the washing. It was an extremely draining schedule, and those days contained very little joy. I'm sure my bad attitude towards the rehab floor didn't help matters. I also had a roommate for the first time since I had been hospitalized, which was aggravating when you're used to having a private room. He was a young construction worker who had fallen a large distance and was paralyzed from the neck down. We talked very little, mostly due to both of our bad attitudes toward our bad situations. Having a roommate also made things challenging when my kids came to visit. Keeping them quiet and not staring at my roommate or any of the other patients on the floor was very difficult, while in a private room this was much less of a problem.

The gym part of the rehab unit was a long thin room with tons of equipment in different sections. This equipment varied from very expensive machines to sets of long parallel bars and large vinyl-covered "beds." Each section was full of different equipment, one section for occupational therapy, one for physical therapy, and the area in the middle was shared by the two. During each hour, each therapist had two or three patients to work with. The therapist had to move between their patients and keep them going on exercises. They often worked with me on exercises where I needed to be worked with one-on-one, then would give me drills or exercises to work on my own while they went to work with another patient. It wasn't overcrowded, but it wouldn't have taken many more patients in there to make it tough to move around. Most of us weren't very mobile so we didn't get in each other's way. I wasn't up to walking all the way over to the gym and back, at least early in my stay, so I would wheel over in my wheelchair, then do a little walking between stations once I was there.

Many therapists played a big role in my recovery. I was so weak from being motionless and on a ventilator for three weeks that I basically had to retrain my muscles to even move. Tami, my physical "terrorist," as she called herself, from the Metro Burn Unit had the daunting task of retraining me to walk. The incredible part about Tami was and continues to be her constant, positive attitude and spunk. She is never at a loss for words, very petite in stature, but strong as an ox. She had to be strong to support my big frame as we slowly progressed towards being able to walk again.

Adrian, my physical therapist on the rehab unit, was totally focused on my balance. I suppose that was because my balance stunk after all the muscle loss and nerve damage I had experienced. These exercises were very annoying and painful. Hold yourself in this position, stand on this awkward round-bottomed platform and not fall over, play catch while standing on the round-bottomed platform..., there seemed to be no end to these crazy and annoying exercises. I started out doing most of these between the parallel bars so I could grab on with my one good arm when I lost my balance. All of these exercises made my legs ache something fierce and I really didn't care for them. I kept suggesting the weights, that was something I had done in the past and would be a productive way to take out my frustrations, but she didn't think I was ready for that yet.

In addition to my overall muscle weakness, I was also suffering from foot-drop, a condition most likely due to chronic pressure on the nerves which supplied my shin muscles, anterior tibialis. This can occur from being in bed for long periods of time and is medically known as critical-care neuropathy. This foot-drop meant that I was incapable of lifting my foot at the ankle to get it prepared for the next step. The only way to get around this foot-drop was to lift my whole leg much higher than usual and swing my leg forward and up so my foot would land on the bottom as it should and not on the end of my toes. This was a major frustration for everyone, especially me, as it made recovery and walking much more difficult.

While I was there, the therapists fit me for some plastic braces to keep my foot perpendicular to my leg. These braces were a big help. Instead of lifting my knee up high and flailing my leg so my foot would swing up, this brace kept my foot up so I wouldn't have to worry about my toes getting caught underneath my foot while I was walking. With the braces, I could walk in a more normal pattern and not expend as much energy. I had the peace of mind that I wasn't going to trip on every step. This was the biggest reason I was able to progress as fast as I did. Once I had the braces, I began seeking out additional chances to work on my walking. The unit had a walking practice which was in addition to my scheduled occupational and physical therapy. I started going to this and just basically took turns walking laps around the gym area. They even had some steps, four steps up to a landing, that I would work on. It is amazing how tiring and difficult it was, but I began to feel better and better about my walking. While the braces were life-savers, having most of your leg surrounded by plastic in the middle of summer was very hot and less than comfortable. There was also the embarrassment and unwanted public attention of wearing them with shorts.

After weeks of work and help from Tami and subsequently Adrian on the rehab unit, I was able to walk reasonably well. After trying all kinds of things to stimulate the nerves that affected my foot-drop, nothing seemed to help. I was very anxious, yet tried to be patient with my feet, hoping and praying the foot-drop would resolve. I also had numbness of the top of my feet and lateral shin from the same nerve damage. This added to my discomfort after working these muscles during therapy.

While my walking progressed, my shoulder felt as if it didn't. It wasn't that I wasn't trying, I just didn't make quick progression with it. My shoulder just throbbed with pain all the time and had such a limited range of motion. I kept trying to imagine swinging a golf club, it didn't seem possible that I would be able to hit a ball more than 20 yards. Jen, my occupational therapist there, kept working with me though, and tried to encourage me.

The occupational therapists had the tough job of dealing with my left shoulder and my skin grafts. A great deal of muscle from my left shoulder was gone, and with no real movement over many weeks the joint became almost completely frozen. When you take my surgical loss of muscle, a frozen joint, and surrounding tightly-stretched skin grafts, I was left with very little movement in my left shoulder. That doesn't mean I didn't have pain, my shoulder ached fiercely both before and after my rehabilitation started. The doctors were never able to figure out a reason why, but fortunately that slowly resolved itself. Jen would stretch my shoulder in every direction to the point of unbearable pain, hold it, let off a little then go again. She also had me doing all kinds of exercises designed to improve my strength, movement and coordination. We did make some increase in range of motion, ten to twelve degrees, while I was there, but that was hardly noticeable in the big scheme of things. My left arm was still pretty useless except when I did things with my hand down at my hip level.

Once I was discharged home, I came back in for outpatient therapy three days a week with Kathy. This is where the real action got going. Kathy was more of a sweet, quiet therapist who could smile so nicely while she stretched my shoulder without mercy. She would do both stretching and graft-massage with me, then set me up with exercises to actively use my shoulder. Every degree of increase in my shoulder range of motion was a victory for us, paid for with our hard work and my pain. Skin grafts, once they take to an area, tend to stick to whatever is beneath them. For maximum mobility around the grafts, the backside of the grafts need to be secondarily loosed from the bone and soft tissue underneath. Massage seems like too nice a word for this task, with lotion and incredible pressure, Kathy slowly mobilized my skin grafts one area at a time. She would also stretch my head away from my left shoulder attempting to stretch the grafts of the left side of my neck. It felt, at times as if my skin was just going to let go and tear open. As tough as this was on me, I know that I have Jen, Kathy and the other occupational therapists to thank for all the function and mobility I have in my left shoulder and neck.

During my stay on the rehab unit, I also was beginning to have a new problem with my donor sites. They were starting to itch to the point that I was aggressively scratching at them. This was worse when I was standing up without moving. It was unbearable at times. The donor sites would turn purple and I would just have to sit down. They tried some different medication to stop the itching, but I found that I couldn't stand still. If I was moving or sitting or lying, they didn't itch too badly, but standing still was unbearable. I'm not sure which was worse, the intense pain post-surgery or the incredible itching these donor sites gave me during this stage. This condition lasted a couple of months before finally easing off. The doctors were never able to figure out why this was happening for sure. I suspect that I had some clots at the filter that had been put in to keep clots from going to my lungs. My theory is that these clots plugged blood flow, more when I was standing still and my muscles weren't pumping to keep the blood moving. This backup of venous blood made the grafts turn purple and stimulated them to itch. Thank goodness that wasn't permanent. A lot of my ailments were temporary, but at the time, no one knew what would happen. I spent a lot of time worrying about what was going to last and what would go away.

During this time, Chase turned two and we were able to have a party in a special children's play area at Metro. Michelle and my mom worked hard to plan a fun party, which everyone enjoyed, especially the kids. This place had all kinds of neat activities for the kids to do in a large windowed annex. I still had a poor appetite, all the party food that I usually loved so much wasn't very appealing.

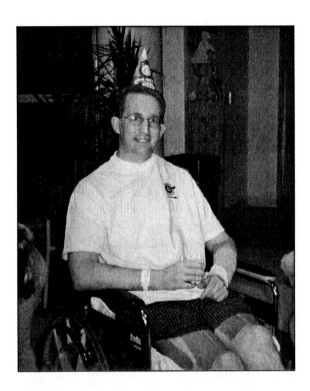

Craig at Chase's 2nd Birthday Party.

Rehabilitation in a general sense is a mixed bag for patients. It is a positive step in the fact that this usually occurs in the recovery phase of an illness and shows progress by the patient. The negative aspect of rehabilitation is the pain that almost always accompanies the hard work it takes to recover the functions of daily living.

As tough as therapy can be, I am living proof of how successful it can be. While going through rehabilitation, things seemed like they would never improve. Progress was painful and painfully slow. With patience, a positive attitude and great therapists almost anything is possible. I distinctly remember lying in my hospital bed, too weak to even sit up, unable to move my left arm, and in significant amounts of pain thinking, "How can I ever get back to my life; walking, running, playing with my kids, golfing, working?" There isn't much need for one-armed pediatricians. Now a full four years later, I am very functional, doing almost everything that seemed unlikely or impossible lying in that hospital bed. While it wasn't easy, the functional abilities I have now more than make up for all the hard work that came before.

2 Corinthians 12:9 "My grace is sufficient for thee: for my strength is made perfect in weakness."

So the days dragged on in the rehab unit. Even though I was unhappy with my situation there, my resolve to get rehabilitated enough to get discharged home was strong and I worked hard trying to improve my walking and balance. I could really taste going home now. I was so tired of being confined to the hospital. As often as I could, I had Michelle or my mom take me downstairs to get something "real" to eat, and whenever the weather was decent we would go outside and sit in a courtyard just outside the cafeteria. This was an especially good idea when the boys were with us so they could run around a little bit. I knew I would have to use the wheelchair a lot when I got home, but I didn't care, I wanted out. Every day I got stronger, although I certainly felt far from strong. Once I had my braces, I felt like I could do it. Sooner than anyone thought possible, I got the OK to be released eight days after being transferred to the rehab unit. All the doctors had predicted two to three weeks so I was very pleased that this was well ahead of schedule. Now a full two months after being admitted to the hospital I was going home. I knew I would have to come back for one more round of surgery, but to get out of the hospital for more than just a few hours was something I had dreamed about for a very long time.

Journal Entry - July 2000

Craig, Michelle and Family:

When you arrived at Metro, nobody knew what the outcome would be. You were very sick and hardly able to maintain a blood pressure with the help of fluids and pressors. After multiple hurdles, surgeries and rehabilitation, you have overcome a great deal. Your faith, courage, strength and determination is an inspiration. Although the road ahead may be rough at times, you have done so much and come so far. Don't ever forget that.

Your recovery not only gives us cause to celebrate as well but reminds us why we do the things we do in our profession. It has been a pleasure caring for you. You are blessed with a wonderful family (all of you). I wish you much happiness with your growing family, new home and success in your practice!

Love and God Bless, AnnMarie G.

Chapter 9

Reprieve

What an exciting trip it was for me, the day I finally got to see the apartment I had heard so much about. I am a very visual person, so I had tried to picture the apartment based on everyone's description, but as is usually the case, it was different than I had imagined. In the section of Lakewood where we were staying, most of the houses were duplexes. Instead of having the units side to side as I was used to, these large houses had one unit above and one unit below. The house we were staying in had a big front porch with a small amount of yard in the front and back. It had a long driveway that went the entire length of the property to a freestanding garage with a basketball hoop in the back corner of the lot. The driveway was about one car-width and equaled the distance between the houses. Behind the house, there was enough parking for one of our vehicles. It was a little dicey getting in and out of the tight space but fortunately we never had any mishaps. Whenever someone was visiting us they had to park on the street along with one of our vehicles. Ryan and Kathy, the owners of the property, had two dalmatians, Otis and Ollie, who were very rambunctious and hard on the yard. To make life easier for themselves and for extra parking, they had mulched and graveled the entire backyard area so the dogs could do their business and not tear up the lawn. In front of the house there was a small patch of grass between the front porch and the sidewalk. It probably took longer to get the lawn mower out, filled with gas and started than it did to mow it.

After two and a half months in the hospital, I was free. I was home and moving back in with Michelle, Taylor, Chase, and my mom, who was still staying with us. It is hard to put into words all the feelings I felt, finally having freedom from the confines of the hospital. I was brimming with anticipation as we pulled into the drive. All those days and nights confined to a hospital bed and room can drive a person crazy. I was finally on my own to do things on my schedule. I was home with my family, my bed and some privacy. Welcome home signs and two excited little boys were there to greet us when we arrived "home."

As wonderful as it was, being at home also put lots of pressure on Michelle. She had to do all the work of care and support for me that was previously done by the nurses and staff in the hospital. This was in addition to her helping my mom cook, clean, and take care of the kids. Michelle was now seven months pregnant, and exhausted by all the stress and sleepless nights from my extended illness. I was able to walk short distances, but I was still wobbly. This was especially true when I didn't have my foot-drop braces on, like when I was in bed. Michelle insisted that she get up and go with me to the bathroom in the middle of the night, she wasn't about to have me fall. More than one person was worried about Michelle and the baby after going through all the stress and exhaustion the previous two months had provided.

Matthew 6:25, 27, 33-34 "Therefore I tell you, do not worry about your life, what you will eat or drink; or about your body, what you will

wear. Is not life more important than food, and the body more important than clothes? Who of you by worrying can add a single hour to
his life? But seek first His kingdom and His righteousness, and all
these things will be given to you as well. Therefore do not worry about
tomorrow, tomorrow will worry about itself. Each day has enough
trouble of its own."

Though neither of us were working, our days were busy,
filled with all the activities associated with my care and the care
of the boys. Everything was a struggle for me. Just getting a bath
or shower was an ordeal. I had limited strength in my left shoulder and not much more anywhere else, so it was hard to get my
big frame into the tub gracefully. There weren't any rails to hold
on to, so I ended up getting down on my hands and knees. Once
I was down, I would slowly roll into the tub. Until you find
yourself in a situation like mine, it is hard to imagine how difficult the simplest daily activities can be. Soon after I was home,
we purchased a Rubbermaid shower chair which helped tremendously. I couldn't stand upright long enough to get my
shower and getting down into the tub was difficult and uncomfortable. The chair had to go long-ways to fit so I didn't have the
benefit of the backrest, but I was sure glad to have something
elevated and stable to sit on in the shower.

After getting out of the shower, Michelle would cover my
wounds with antibiotic ointment, then some yellow Vaseline
gauze known as Xeroform. Then came regular gauze followed
by ace bandages to keep the dressings in place. All those layers
were very hot in the middle of the summer. The guaze and ace
bandages had to go around my neck on the left side in order for
them not to slide down, so all these bulky bandages were not the
picture of comfort. It also made one shoulder appear higher than
the other, but there was nothing that could be done about it. Between the braces on my skinny chicken legs, candy-cane stripes

on my thighs from my donor sites, bandages on my left forearm and a lopsided hunchback, passers by had plenty to stare at. Out of necessity, Michelle became very adept at all the nursing activities needed to keep me going at home.

Speaking of nursing duties, the part of our daily routine that I hated the most had to be getting my Lovenox shot. Michelle had been taught by the nurses to give me the shot at home once a day. The medicine was prescribed to prevent more blood clots in my legs and worsening of the ones I already had. After the thousands of pokes I had gone through already, you would think that one little shot per day wouldn't be too bad, but this particular shot was awful. Wherever the shot was given to me, it felt like I had a blow torch going wide open on my skin for a good five minutes. It was somewhat similar to getting lidocaine, the medicine used to numb an area on our body before stiches or other painful procedures. The big difference was that this extreme burning lasted five minutes instead of five seconds with the lidocaine. The lidocaine is acidic and that is the part of that injection that hurts the worst. I assume the Lovenox is bad for the same reason. The best place we found to give it to me was right along the grafts on my stomach. Some of the patches of real skin along the grafts were very numb which helped make the shot bearable. We didn't know whether we were in a good area or not until the needle went through the skin. After having it many times, I was able to figure out areas that had the best chance of numbness and tried to steer Michelle in that direction as much as possible. These good areas became hard and bruised so we were forced to use the more painful areas as time went on.

As with all the things I didn't like during my illness, I tried to negotiate my way out of these Lovenox shots. Every time I saw the doctors, I tried to convince them I didn't need them anymore. I felt well protected with my vena cava filter in to keep any blood clots from coming up from my legs to my lungs, and I was getting more active everyday. Dr. Fratianne and Yowler both held their ground though, they were worried I would get phlebitis if I didn't keep my blood "thinned." The clots were still present on my ultrasound, so, that was that. I kept telling them I was willing to take the chance, but they made it clear they weren't.

Michelle wasn't budging on it either. She knew what the doctors were saying and wasn't interested in any type of problem for me. "I almost lost you once, I'm not going to do anything to jeopardize you now." I can just hear her saying that, especially since I have continued to hear it ever since. I kept trying to play my doctor card, that I knew what I was talking about and didn't really need the shots but Michelle didn't buy it. She would stop giving me the shot where it hurt the least when that area started to get discolored and hardened. Michelle didn't trust my medical judgement when it came to my own personal care anymore. She wasn't about to let me talk her out of anything again, not like I had when I convinced her to go home from the hospital the night my ordeal began.

The inside of our portion of the apartment consisted of a small kitchen, a large dining area, a large living room, two small bedrooms and a small bathroom. Down one floor in the basement was a washer and dryer that we shared with Ryan and Kathy. Our place was furnished with only the bare essentials, most of our belongings had already been moved to Pennsylvania. Our dining room table was a flimsy, portable table that Michelle's parents had lent to us. It was one they often used while they were camping. We also had folding chairs to sit on and folding lawn chairs in the living room. I jokingly call these folding chairs we used at the table in the dining room my "favorites." They look like small director's chairs and I always pinched my fingers whenever I tried to open and close them. The canvas back was so small and low it was impossible to lean back on them at all, making them uncomfortable. In both bedrooms there were mattresses and box springs on the floor without their frames. The only other large piece of furniture we had in the apartment was a recliner that Michelle's parents had brought from Pennsylvania for me to use. I needed a place to be somewhat comfortable and the lawn chairs didn't cut it, especially with my armpit wound still open in back. The chairs didn't work well for anybody else either, but they had to make the best of it.

Sleeping at home was just as difficult as it was for me in the hospital. In one way it was worse, now I had Michelle lying next me, who I was trying hard not to disturb. Before my illness I had slept with my left arm under my pillow, lying on my stomach. My left arm was difficult to move without pain and getting it bent up under my pillow was out of the question, so my choices were to lie flat on my back or on my right side. What sleep I did have was very restless, and I changed positions frequently trying to find a comfortable one. I continued sleeping only one-to-two hours at a time as I had been doing in the hospital. Our bedroom in the apartment had an air-conditioner in the window which had to go full blast to cool the whole apartment. This kept it very cold in our room, which made it undesirable to be outside the covers. I did fine with the constant noise though, and this helped to drown out the noise of trains as they went by several times a night. The tracks were only a distance of about ten houses from ours, so we all knew when they were going by. The whole sleeping situation was a challenge to get used to. I just wasn't sleeping regularly yet. Michelle wasn't sleeping very well either due to her bulging belly. Often, I would get so uncomfortable in bed I would go out to the recliner to get a new position and give Michelle a couple hours of uninterrupted sleep.

Since there wasn't much room for the kids to play outside at the apartment, Michelle and my mom had checked out the west-side area for some parks. We were fortunate that there were several possibilities within a very short distance of our house. I had heard about the different parks during visits from my mom and Michelle, and I was especially interested to see the lakefront park that they had gone to several times. For those of you that don't know, Cleveland sits right on Lake Erie, one of the Great Lakes. On the east side of town where we had lived, the lakefront parks where further east, so seeing the lake was not a common thing for us. The shoreline east of downtown was dominated by an airport and expensive homes. After being in the hospital for so long, I had a very strong desire to get out and see the lake, especially since I had been hearing so much about it. The first time we went, I didn't feel like I was strong enough to walk the entire way from the car to the lake so we tried to do it in the wheelchair. The park had a large, grassy area full of little bumps and ruts. It was a bouncy ride and was very difficult for Michelle to push me through. The tough ride was well worth it though. The park comes up to the edge of a bluff overlooking the lake, opening up to an incredible view. Looking to the east from the bluff, it was easy to see the high-rises of downtown. Our stay there was very peaceful as we watched the small waves lap onto the shore, and the sailboats and speedboats cruise around. I have always loved lakes after spending lots of my early years at my grandparent's lake house in Michigan. I remember lots of swimming, boating and fishing, and sitting there brought back lots of good memories. Thinking is something I do a great deal of, so I enjoyed the opportunity to think in a beautiful setting like this. With all that had gone on in the last few months of my life, I had plenty to think about. I couldn't spend all the time thinking though, we had two little boys scurrying around who I was worried would go over the bluff into the lake. During our stay in Lakewood, we made several trips back, but each of these times I walked to the lake. It was definitely the lesser of two evils.

Shortly after I was discharged from the hospital, Michelle's parents came to visit, then took the boys with them back to Pennsylvania. As they were leaving, my mom also left and traveled to North Carolina for my cousin's wedding, then home to Mississippi for the first time since I had taken ill. As a result, Michelle and I had a week together in the apartment by ourselves. It was a good week, a chance for Michelle and me to be together without the children, something we hadn't really done in the four years since Taylor was born. Looking back, we wish I would have felt better and had the strength to doing more things, but the dressing change and rehabilitation schedule kept me pretty exhausted. I spent most of my home time resting or sleeping in the recliner. I was still in a significant amount of pain as well from the open defect in my back and armpit. Despite these hardships, it was good for us, we had some quiet time to talk about things without the interruptions of the hospital or kids. We had so many feelings we needed to get out. Our emotions were strong from all we'd been through, yet I was still somewhat numb in regards to my true feelings. There was the joy of being home, yet I still had plenty of anger for mine and everyone else's suffering, fear of not knowing how much function I would recover, disappointment on not being able to graduate on time or start my new job, and frustration from my physical limitations, pain, and continued weakness. Michelle was contrastingly so joyful about my recovery, I think it was hard for her to deal with some of my fouler moods. She often asked me if my feelings had changed about her through our ordeal. It was hard for me to return her affection, mostly due to the discomfort any type of pressure caused on my grafts and donor sites. Every hug was painful for me, so while I loved the affection, it came with a price. Acting is not one of my strengths, so she easily knew when I was hurting. Understandably, she sometimes misconstrued my discomfort as a sign that I didn't want that affection. Her emotions were running high and pregnancy hormones were raging. It took Michelle a while to come to peace with my difficulty showing and receiving affection. Fortunately, the whole situation improved over time. Our relationship renewed and grew stronger by the day as I felt better and as she saw that I was still totally in love with her.

My state of mind was one of constant change. Some moments were full of joy at my release from the hospital, some were hard as I felt sorry for myself because of my horrible scarring and continued pain in my left shoulder. The status of my faith at that point is hard to pin down. For the majority of my hospitalization, I was more numb to my feelings than anything else. There were brief spells of anger and sadness, but mostly I was in survival mode. My brain, which is usually pumping out constant thoughts of this and that seemed more in a quiet, power-save mode. A couple of times in the hospital, Michelle wanted to read to me from the journal that she had been keeping, but I resisted. Like many men, I hated crying and always tried to avoid situations where that might happen. The few times she did read to me from the journal, I really broke down. As I heard the words of my friends and family from the time period when my life hung in the balance, I couldn't contain the sadness and tears. Michelle saw this as healthy, I just didn't want to face it and lose control of my emotions. Now that I was home, I found myself feeling more anger and got into that questioning mode. "Why did this happen to me? What did I do to deserve it? Was God punishing me or did he just look away, allowing the devil to do this awful thing?" My emotions were continually bouncing between being thankful for surviving an almost uniformly lethal-infection and being upset that I had to go through such a horrible experience in the first place. Now I was scarred and basically useless to do anything productive. All our plans were on hold, our finances were in the toilet and I had no idea what kind of function I would recover. How were we ever going to really recover from this? Had our unborn baby been harmed from going through all the stress Michelle had endured? Looking back, I think all these questions and concerns were part of any normal course of recovery from such a devastating illness.

Michelle was trying to get me to see the positive, from her standpoint she was overjoyed that I had overcome the infection and all its complications, even though my body was significantly scarred. It was an ironic situation for us, she is usually the pessimist, though she would say realist, trying to bring the optimist in me back down to earth. She was disappointed in my discouragement but did her best to understand and accept it. Her prayers had been answered so it was hard for her to see my struggling faith as I started over with my changed life. She was determined to help me see what a miracle my recovery was and look for the positives in it. While Michelle had a strong faith prior to my illness, she had grown to a whole new level in response to my recovery. She had witnessed the very miracle she had prayed so hard for.

My faith in God was shaken but not destroyed by my illness. I still believed in God and prayed to him for healing. Despite this, I was not ready to admit that my suffering could somehow be for good. I was far from being able to forgive God for allowing these "flesh-eating" bacteria to ravage my body and turn our entire world upside down. I couldn't deny that Michelle and others close to me had seen their faith strengthened, I just failed to see why I deserved this fate or deserved to suffer for the betterment of others. I know Jesus did this for us and that I should be willing to do it for my loved ones, but I wasn't there yet. The old saying goes "whatever doesn't kill you makes you stronger." During this reprieve from the hospital, I certainly didn't feel stronger. I wasn't depressed and despite my anger and grieving for my former body, I was trying to channel this energy into getting better so we could get things wrapped up in Cleveland and move on to Pennsylvania. I was hoping my attitude would improve in new surroundings. Having concrete goals was always a good thing for me.

After discussing the idea during the week, we decided it would be beneficial for all of us to get away from the city, to travel to Pennsylvania to see our extended family, our new house, and pick up the boys at Grammy and Pappy's. This would give me a reprieve from the therapy routine for a four-day weekend. My mom returned from Mississippi just in time to go along with us. We debated whether or not I was strong enough to make the trip, but I really felt it would do me good, at least spiritually. The trip from Cleveland to Pennsylvania takes about four hours, depending on traffic and construction, which is a given on Interstate 80 in the summer. Just like shorter car trips, the bumps and jarring of the wound on the back of my shoulder was very painful. Since this was a longer car ride, I was extremely sore and tired when we arrived in Pennsylvania. Despite the discomfort, I felt triumphant and overjoyed to be away from the city and hospital, if only for a short period. It was strange being the passenger instead of the driver, one of the many role reversals we had endured since my illness.

Staying at Michelle's parent's house was another new challenge. They had more steps in their house than in our apartment. The steps are polished hardwood so I was scared I would slip on them and fall down the steps. I figured out that it was better to put my shoes and braces on before tackling the steps, especially before descending. I felt so clumsy and off-balance on flat surfaces that anything else made me really nervous. I was using a cane to help my balance but I didn't feel comfortable using it on the steps either. I just took things at a slow and careful pace and fortunately had no accidents.

While we were there, we had a big birthday party to celebrate Taylor's turning four. All of Michelle's family came for a big picnic, it was nice to see everyone. I was pretty self-conscious of how I looked, all scarred and thin, but I tried hard not to worry about it. It was difficult not to think about it as people's eyes wandered to my scars on my arm, legs and neck, still fire engine red. This was family and they knew what I had been through, unlike people who would see me on the street.

Before I got sick, we had decided to get Taylor his first two-wheeled bike with training wheels for his big birthday present. It needed to be assembled so Michelle's dad had done it in my absence. Although there was nothing I could do about it, it did leave me feeling guilty that I couldn't physically do this important thing for him. Michelle's dad is an expert in everything mechanical so Taylor probably lucked out in a sense that his bike got put together better than if I would have assembled it. Taylor was so excited to get the bike and ride it that the feelings of guilt and self-pity went by the wayside quickly. These feelings of worthlessness would emerge now and then as time went on. It was tough going from the important, strong and capable dad to an incapable, weak drain on our family's resources. I did my best to use these feelings of self-pity as motivation to get better.

While we were in Pennsylvania, we were able to see our new house and restore in our minds what everything there looked like. Things were pretty overgrown. Michelle's dad and grandfather had kept the yard mowed, in addition to mowing their own yards, but all the bushes were trying to take over the place. Inside the house, things were scattered all around and the dust and grime were evident, but we knew we would love living there once we got it in shape. Our old stone house was so unique and full of history and character. Most of our furniture was there and Michelle's parents had already started unpacking many of the boxes the movers had brought in. How I wished I could stay there, not having to go back to Cleveland for a final surgery, and one last month of residency. It was tempting to just stay and consider us moved, but we had some unfinished business back across the state line.

Along with seeing lots of friends and family, I was also able to go and visit my soon-to-be doctor colleagues and give them an update on my status. I think it was good for them to see all the progress I had made. I was also able to see my desk and reaffirm how happy I was with my new practice choice. Although going back to Cleveland was tough, seeing everyone and everything we were working towards was really good for me, helping my spirit to stay positive during the final stretch of my recovery. After a wonderful four days with friends and family, we headed back to Cleveland to continue my therapy prior to my upcoming surgery.

Once we were back at our apartment in Cleveland, we resumed our routine of daily dressing changes and frequent trips to the hospital for therapy and doctor's visits. As my strength improved, we began to venture out a little more frequently, to do some shopping or to go out to eat. For the entire time I was awake in the hospital and even at this point, I didn't have the greatest appetite. That was finally starting to pick up. I was such a bean pole, so when my appetite started returning I was ready to eat some good food. We started to go to all of my favorite restaurants whenever I had the energy and we could fit it in. I had been given strict instructions to push calories wherever I could to try to regain some of the weight I had lost, so I gave it my best shot. Even when I felt really hungry, I would start eating then hit a wall where I couldn't eat another bite. We were taking home lots of doggie bags, which prior to my illness was a rare thing for me. I had never had trouble finishing a meal.

It was during this time in the apartment that I got my first good look at my "new" body. For so long, I didn't have the opportunity since I was always bandaged. I had seen my donor sites on my legs and arm but that was it. I had been too weak to get my head off the spray table during my dressing changes. Even after I had the strength to stretch and see my scars, I had

115

no desire to look. I can't explain why. Maybe it was the fear of what I looked like, but I just didn't have any desire to know. I suppose it was my subconscious denial-stage of grieving for my former body. Then it happened, I saw myself, by accident, in the mirror after getting out of the shower one day. I remember the total surprise, followed by feelings of disgust at how awful I looked. I guess I had unconsciously been blocking my visualizing mind, not even attempting to guess what my skin grafts and donor sites looked like. The grafts were vividly red, contrasting the pale skin surrounding them. My left chest was mostly gone, with a little patch of skin including my nipple remaining. My left nipple was now much closer to my sternum than the right one. My belly was another peninsula of normal skin surrounded by a sea of red, only now my belly button was noticeably pushed to the right. Above my left collarbone I had this large concave hole big enough to put your fist in. Not only did I have all the scars, I was a bean pole, all skin and bones. It didn't look like me at all. I wasn't anything special to look at before, but now..., I was ugly with a capital U, grotesque. The Six-Million Dollar Man had sure looked better than this. It was going to take some time to adjust to this new body. The most positive thing I could come up with was that most of my scars would be covered with clothing. Michelle assured me that she didn't care, she was so glad to have whatever was left of me around. How lucky I was in that sense, looking the way I did would have been a big obstacle had I been single, searching for a mate. My friends and family didn't shun me because of how I looked. What did it really matter? I had a new appreciation for all people with distorted bodies and disabilities. While having all this scarring wasn't pleasant, I was never so concerned about body image before getting sick that I couldn't deal with it now. I know there are plenty of people in this world with worse scarring than I had. I had seen them on the job as a doctor and right there in the burn unit. I also knew that I, Craig Harold Collison, was much more than flesh and bones. I had a spirit that was the true me, that would live on even when this body was history. In spite of knowing this, I knew I had to deal with this body for the rest of my earthly life, so I started down the road of accepting my scars.

Chapter 10

Final Reconstruction

I had mixed emotions going into my last surgery. It was now mid-July and the time to go under the knife again had come. Part of me was scared, not looking forward to another round of anesthesia, intubation, surgery and post-surgical pain. I was feeling better all the time, and I knew the surgery would reverse that trend, even if only temporarily. Having worked so hard to get to this point in my recovery, the thought of even a small setback was disheartening. The other part of me was ready, ready to get in and get everything over with sooner rather than later. I had the taste of freedom from the hospital and was now focused on a full recovery, so we could move forward. Would this be my final surgery, or another setback? Would I be well enough to start my residency rotation at the beginning of August? These questions weighed heavily on all of us as the date approached for this next hurdle.

𝔓𝔥𝔦𝔩𝔩𝔦𝔭𝔦𝔞𝔫𝔰 4:13 "𝔍 𝔠𝔞𝔫 𝔡𝔬 𝔞𝔩𝔩 𝔱𝔥𝔦𝔫𝔤𝔰 𝔱𝔥𝔯𝔬𝔲𝔤𝔥 𝔆𝔥𝔯𝔦𝔰𝔱 𝔴𝔥𝔬 𝔤𝔦𝔳𝔢𝔰 𝔪𝔢 𝔰𝔱𝔯𝔢𝔫𝔤𝔱𝔥."

As is normal procedure prior to anesthesia and surgery, I was not allowed to eat or drink anything after midnight the night prior to my surgery. This is always difficult for every patient awaiting surgery, and was even worse for me since my surgery wasn't scheduled to start until 1:00 PM. While I wasn't back to a normal appetite by any stretch of the imagination, that morning I was uncomfortable in my stomach from both hunger and nervous butterflies. As if 1:00 wasn't late enough, my surgery was bumped due to other surgeries going longer than expected, all completely out of my surgeon's control. This pushed the start time for my surgery back to 3:30 p.m.; two and a half extra hours of torture, lying in bed in only a gown, one foot from the next patient who was playing the same waiting game I was. Michelle was great, doing her best to keep my mind as occupied as possible. She was always so positive and strong, at least in front of me. Her mental toughness during my entire illness was unlike anything I'd seen from her. It was a definite role reversal for us. Michelle, now less than a month away from her pregnancy due date and two months into this life-changing episode, was so strong and courageous. She could have lost it, withdrawn, or felt sorry for herself, but she stood up to the challenge better than anyone would have expected. I attribute this to her faith, giving her spirit the strength to persevere and believe in my miraculous recovery.

The surgery involved skin grafting a few patches around my full-thickness graft in my armpit, trying to definitively close the last parts of the massive hole left by the flesh-eating bacteria. The full-thickness graft they had taken from my left forearm was well healed now, so Dr. Fratianne and Dr. Kaufman felt better attaching new grafts to it with sutures and staples. Having been through so much, I was praying hard that these grafts would take and this chapter in my recovery would be over. Since everything about my particular case was unique, the surgeons had no idea if the grafts would be strong enough to keep my skin closed and give me some mobility in my left shoulder. I was about ninety percent closed up prior to the surgery and I was ready to get the final ten percent over with. Unfortunately, there was no guarantee this would work.

The surgery itself went fine, without any complications. They took more grafts from my leg and from across my lower back to supply the skin they needed to close everything up. After a couple hours of surgery and a short stay in post-operative recovery, I was taken back to my old room on the step-down part of the burn unit.

One of the most amazing things about the final surgery was how much less pain I had immediately after it was over. On one of my visits back to Rainbow and University Hospitals, Dr. Goldstein had told me that I would feel a lot better once my wounds were completely closed up, and he was right. Having open wounds for a long period of time was very uncomfortable, and just getting them surgically closed would supposedly make me feel much better. Even as I was waking up from my surgery, I couldn't believe the dramatic reduction in the pain in back of my armpit. I had discomfort from my new donor sites, but from the moment I awoke I felt tremendously better than I had since my illness began. The constant ache radiating from the back of my left shoulder was gone. I had only one dose of pain medication after I was awakened, and I'm not sure I needed it. I agreed to it thinking the pain would increase as the anesthesia wore off but it never did. This was an incredible blessing to me, that I actually felt better after all the manipulation, cutting, stapling, and suturing I had just been through.

My shoulder was immobilized with a large, padded sling which held my upper arm straight down my side and my forearm across my stomach. I could move my fingers but that was all the movement I had. I felt so good when I got to my room after surgery, I decided I could handle some apple juice. The nurses warned me to take it slow, but I was so thirsty and dry in my throat from having a breathing tube in that I chugged it right down. While it felt great going down, I instantly got nauseated and vomited it right back up. Then I was fine again. I was a little embarrassed and didn't want to tell the nurses that I had thrown up and hear "I told you so," so I just left the little basin there. I'm sure they must have figured me out since someone had to dump it later. I learned an important lesson, that anesthesia is hard on the stomach and taking things slowly right after surgery is smart, even if you are feeling pretty good.

My next few days were pretty uneventful, waiting for the day when they would unwrap me and see how my grafts were healing. I was back in the same room I had been in previously on the less acute part of the burn unit, so it was nice to feel better than I had the first time I was in there. This room didn't have a nice view like my room on the critical side. There was another building about ten feet from my window. Unfortunately, this room had an old fuzzy TV with the same limited selection as before. On the wall, the room had a surreal impressionist painting of flowers, much more peaceful than the battle scene from my first room. The room was right by the front door of the unit, so the secretaries were right there. With everyone coming in and out there, it was noisy and busy most of the time. This room was also positioned right under the transport helicopter pad so it shook every time the helicopter took off and landed. We could even smell exhaust fumes from the helicopter in my room, presumably through the air intakes. I was able to get around better now that I had my foot-drop braces, but I mostly stayed in bed. While my shoulder felt better than it had in months, my new donor sites were sore. Since there were only two sites, I could protect them better than when I had them all over my legs and back. It was a challenge sleeping or doing anything with my left arm completely strapped to my body. I felt off-balance when I did get up. It was just easier overall to stay in bed. I got up to use the bathroom and that was about it.

Three days after my surgery, the big unwrapping took place. My family and I were anxious to hear how well the grafts had taken and whether or not it looked like my surgeries were over. The whole procedure felt like a "Chinese fire drill," with a large crowd of people stuffed into my little room. All these doctors and nurses were there, crawling over one another removing the layers of bandages and surveying the work. It didn't hurt as badly as the first time I had gone through a major unwrapping, but all the pulling and tugging didn't feel the greatest either. After surveying their work, everyone was pleased. Dr. Fratianne thought the findings were good, the grafts looked healthy and seemed to be covering all the open areas. I was all patched up, at least for the moment. I was re-wrapped and the routine of daily dressing changes started again. During the last few days of my final stay in the burn unit, the therapists started doing some gentle, passive range of motion with my left shoulder. They had to take things extremely slow so as not to disrupt the fresh grafts. They also knew that my shoulder needed to get moving again so I wouldn't lose all the range of motion I had achieved prior to my surgery.

I stayed in the hospital for a total of eight days while they monitored my progress. Things went well, without any big setbacks. The surgery's apparent success was a huge blessing for all of us. It was special going home again, this time, we hoped, for good. No more sleeping in the hospital, getting interrupted every few hours for vital signs, no more blood draws or IV's, no more hospital food. I still had lots of recovering to do but I was ready for it. I had less than a week to get myself strong enough to start my behavioral rotation.

Journal Entry - July 2000

Dr. Collison, Michelle and Family:

We are very thankful for your recovery. We watched you and cared for you from your critical status, now recovery. It is a pleasure seeing your progress. The important things now are to watch you grow and meet the challenges that are ahead of you. I think of the many patients that will be inspired by you. There will be many times that you will not even know about...

If you ever wonder about the purpose and reasons for your suffering, just know that for some reason this is preparing you for the future and God only knows what that involves. Remember, you are always part of our family. If you think of us on the Burn team, think of us as being motivated and inspired by you. Take care - Be great and keep in touch.

Lynne Y. RN

Chapter 11

Resurfacing

Psalm 34:4 "I sought the Lord, and He answered me; He delivered me from all my fears. Those who look to him are radiant, their faces are never covered in shame."

A rriving back at the apartment for the second time, we knew we had a busy month to work through in August. Along with my residency requirements, we were expecting the baby to arrive sometime that month. On top of all this, we had to figure out how we were going to get all of us and the rest of our belongings to Penn-

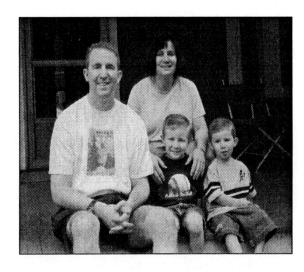

Craig, Michelle, Taylor and Chase on the front porch of our apartment in Cleveland.

sylvania. I continued to need daily dressing changes at home and I was doing physical and occupational therapy four days a week back at Metro, it wasn't going to be easy. Luckily, we were excited about all these events. Finishing my residency, having a new baby, getting my body stronger and preparing to move to Pennsylvania were all positive things, closing some chapters and starting many new ones in our lives.

The topic of resurfacing is something I would not have thought about had I not gone through my illness experience. I found it very challenging to resurface, to see countless people I knew well, before going through such a traumatic time. While on a different scale, I believe the feeling is similar to a soldier coming back from war. These soldiers see so much devastation and endure such emotional trauma, many war veterans have trouble talking about their experiences to those who haven't experienced it. This can be classified as an illness known as PTSD, Post Traumatic Stress Disorder. I found it extremely difficult to talk about my illness. What do you say when people come up to you and ask you what it is like to be a miracle? I was still smack in the middle of this life-changing experience and felt uncomfortable talking to others in detail about all the pain and suffering I had endured. How could they possibly understand? How could Michelle, who had been at my side the entire time, even truly empathize with my pain and permanent disfigurement? The word miracle still makes me feel uncomfortable. I never know what to say. If I agree with that statement, it almost comes across as conceited. Disagreeing isn't really an option either, there was no doubt that the very fact I was alive at this point had beaten all the odds. I was basically left speechless when this came up, but my personal quandary bothered Michelle. She wanted me to use the opportunity to give testimony to God's great work in my survival. I could logically see that His hand had been there to guide me through this perilous experience, yet I was still angry with God because I had gone through the whole ordeal in the first place. It's Dr. Frat's classic "state of mind," is your glass half empty or half full? He liked to talk about this. I heard it countless times, most frequently when I was feeling down about my situation. My thoughts and feelings waffled back and forth a great deal. I just tried to let the conversation move on when the miracle thing came up.

Another big struggle I had returning to a regular life was figuring out how hard and fast to push myself with work and other activities. My illness came at such a difficult time, right at the end of my residency with our house sold, our next house already purchased, and without any source of income if I wasn't working. I felt this self-induced pressure to get well quickly. I needed to be well fast, to finish my residency so we could move. Only then could I start working and making money. While we weren't on the verge of homelessness, our finances were stretched beyond our means from seven years of training. During medical school, we only had Michelle's teaching income and my large school loans to live on. During residency we did a little better with my income, but we were just barely squeaking by. Michelle was no longer working outside the home so we didn't have her income to supplement mine. We had some credit card debt, and since I had been ill things were only getting worse. On my reduced disability-income and our "double" house payment since May, we were not making ends meet. We knew we would be okay once I started in practice and our income increased, but we were trying not to dig any bigger a hole than we had to.

I hated feeling like I wasn't doing my share, so once we moved and I started working, I pushed quickly to carry my share of the workload. I had originally been scheduled to begin work at the beginning of July, and this start date was pushed back only two months, which is remarkable considering I was in the hospital two and a half months. I was fortunate to have some elective time left in my residency, which didn't need to be made up, and I was well enough to do my last residency requirement in August. Again, I was fortunate that this was a behavior rotation with no call requirements and enough flexibility to allow my continued rehabilitation. Recovering from such a devastating illness takes time. It was probably a good year before I could say my energy level was one hundred percent. To this day some four years later, my left shoulder continues to slowly improve in strength and flexibility.

If I can give any advice on resurfacing after a long illness, it would be to make time for your recovery whenever possible. I quickly stopped my active rehabilitation as the other responsibilities mounted, which slowed me in regaining my left arm-function. Taking more time for cardiovascular exercise, and strengthening my left arm would have been helpful, but I jumped with both feet into work and home and lost that time for myself. Looking back, a slower start at work would have been smarter. Given our situation though, I believe it was the way it had to be. Everyone's situation is different, so you have to do what is right and needs to be done given your physical limitations. Rest, continued rehabilitation, good nutrition, personal support from loved ones and friends and a "healing spirit" are the key ingredients to successfully resurfacing into the real world.

Once I was home from the hospital for the final time, my mom needed to head back to Mississippi. As a school teacher, she needed to get her room ready for the start of school in the second week of August. She'd given up her summer break to help us out. No one could have known that she was to spend her entire summer with us, but she did it without question. Having her with us brought so many blessings. She got to spend lots of time with her grandsons. I benefited as well, for without her presence, my only visitors in the hospital would've been Michelle and only when she could bring in both kids. Once I was out of the hospital, Taylor and Chase would've had to go to all of my doctor's and therapy appointments as we didn't have any babysitters. We can't ever thank mom enough for her sacrifice. Making sacrifices for your children is part of being a parent, and even with her child at age thirty, she gave up her whole summer to help us through our difficult situation. It wasn't easy for her, being away from Dad and home so much, and keeping up with two busy little boys. We are not sure how we could have done it without her.

The big key for Michelle and me now that mom was leaving was whether or not I was up to driving. I didn't have any doubt that I could handle it, but everyone else seemed nervous. With me driving again, I would be able to go to all my lectures and appointments by myself, sparing Michelle and the boys many hours in the car. Things worked out that my mom had been able to be there until I was strong enough to drive. As terrible as this whole ordeal was, the course we took could have been much worse. We knew that to be the case and we were very thankful for any positives that came out of our experience.

I gave driving a try right before my first lecture back at Rainbow. Michelle and mom were both nervous that I wouldn't be strong enough to handle it, but I had it all worked out in my mind. You really hit a man hard if you take away his ability to drive and I was ready to stop being the passenger all of the time. Our car had a manual transmission, so the trick was to steer with my weak left arm while I shifted with my right. I couldn't keep my left arm up high, so I had to hold on to the bottom of the steering wheel with my left hand while I shifted with my right. Pushing the clutch also felt funny because of the foot-drop and the because of the braces I had on my feet. It didn't take long to get the hang of it again. All the driving went smoothly as long as I was sure not to get caught shifting while I was making a turn. I needed both hands to get the steering wheel rotated enough.

August seemed to creep by. I felt exhausted all the time, running to lectures across town at Rainbow and keeping my regular rehabilitation schedule. Michelle's due date was August 12th, my birthday, but we figured she would go late, just like she had done with her first two pregnancies. I was nervous about being so far away from the hospital with this being Michelle's third baby. We were dependent on Michelle's parents to drive four hours to babysit the boys for us, so I was very concerned we wouldn't have enough time for all this to happen if the baby decided to come fast. Our friends, the Shevock's, were our in-town backups, but as we got to our due date they had to leave because of a death in their family, so we were basically stuck. I think we could have found someone if we were desperate but we didn't have any other friends left in town that knew the kids well enough. My anxiousness made dealing with our somewhat crazy circumstances difficult. Every time Michelle had a contraction, I wanted to call her parents in Pennsylvania and get them headed towards Cleveland. She had lots of contractions, known as Braxton-Hicks contractions, over the two weeks prior to the baby's delivery, so this was a frequent topic of conversation. The contractions got so bad once, we did call and her parents drove in from Pennsylvania. It ended up being a false alarm and her parents headed back to Pennsylvania to continue working at their jobs as long as possible. We felt very bad that they had made the long trip and hoped that the labor would be real the next time we called them to come.

Michelle's true labor started around 1 AM on August 16th and at 6 AM she called her parents again. Michelle worked her way into a contraction pattern of one every five or six minutes, which dragged on through most of the day. Her parents had safely arrived and later in the afternoon I finally convinced her that we needed to go to the hospital. I felt so relieved once we stepped foot into MacDonald House, the women's hospital of University Hospitals. Michelle wanted to get her cervix checked to see how far along she was but didn't want to be admitted and forced to lie in bed until she absolutely had to. Our midwife was unavailable at that point to check her so we had to make a choice, either be admitted or hang out at the hospital and wait. Michelle really wanted to wait so we had dinner at the hospital and then went up to the pediatric resident's lounge, one of my hangouts, to wait. As the evening went on, Michelle was getting exhausted and frustrated that her contractions were not progressing any faster. About 9 PM on the 16th, I convinced her that we should get things checked. When they did check her, she was 6 cm dilated, so she still had 4 cm to go. Michelle really wanted this to go like Chase's delivery, having him naturally, one hour after arriving at the hospital. This was not to be the case. After spending two hours in her hospital bed, she had no change in her cervix now almost 20 hours into her active labor. She was tired and frustrated, the third baby was supposed to be easier than this. It was at this point that Michelle agreed to an epidural and pitocin, a medicine to increase contractions, to help things along. After everything was in place, Carol, our midwife, suggested we both take a nap to rest and let things progress. Given my condition, I was exhausted even though I wasn't the one having contractions. This hour-long nap was really good for both of us. When she was checked again, she was a complete 10 cm dilated and ready to start pushing. At 12:21 AM on August 17th, 2000, Caroline Faith Collison was born after 24 grueling hours of labor. She was 8 pounds, 3 ounces, a full pound bigger than either of the boys. No wonder things went so slowly. We were exhausted but ecstatic to have a healthy baby, and the fact that she was a girl was even more special. By history, Collison's seem to have a higher percentage of boys so I was expecting to have another one. We all had thoughts in the back of our minds about what effects the stresses of everything that we had been through might have had on the baby, but Caroline was born without any signs of trouble. The long labor had taken its toll on both of us, but the wonderful result was well worth the exhaustion.

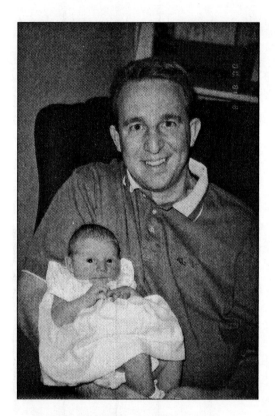

Craig holding Caroline at three days of age in our apartment.

Caroline and Michelle both did great in the hospital and were discharged on August 18th, 36 hours after her birth. Once we were all home, we just had a couple weeks until we were ready to move. My dad flew in from Mississippi, both to see Caroline and to help us get packed. Michelle and the kids headed to Pennsylvania on their own a few days before the end of the month, leaving me alone with dad as I finished my residency requirements. My dad flew back to Mississippi after helping me pack the last remaining items. Michelle's dad and her uncle Kevin then drove over from Pennsylvania with a pickup truck and trailer to help us get the last of our belongings. As is typical when we move, it rained most of the way back to Pennsylvania. Fortunately, they had also brought tarps so our things stayed dry, for the most part. I drove the Mazda back, following the truck and trailer to our house in Pennsylvania. Just after arriving there, a big storm was brewing so we hurriedly got everything inside. At last we were there. Knowing our difficult situation, six ladies from our home church, Fairbrook United Methodist, had spent a day cleaning our house prior to having everything moved in. This was such a blessing for us since we didn't have the capabilities to do that. We knew that it would be months before we had everything in place, but the big move was done and we had made it permanently to Pennsylvania. We had Labor Day weekend to get ourselves somewhat settled before I started work on Tuesday. I was exhausted, which was a permanent state for me as I tried to regain strength, start working, and help out a little at home. While we had made it through the most terrible experience in our lives, we were far from being back to "normal." With a newborn infant, a dad who was weak and frail and a house filled with boxes, we had a long way to go. Despite our tough situation, the events of the previous months had been much worse and we met this next challenge head-on with all the energy we could muster.

Epilogue

The many transitions we experienced after our move to Pennsylvania were both exciting and exhausting. I began working as a Pediatrician on September 5th, the day after Labor Day. While my first month consisted of only half-days, this schedule was more than enough as I tried to rebuild my strength. I was fortunate in that I didn't have many problems doing my job because of my physical ailments. My biggest struggle was getting my left-hand up high enough on bigger kids to pull back their ear as I looked in with my otoscope. Pulling on the earlobe helps straighten the ear canal and makes it easier to see the eardrum. I could have had all these patients lie down but I was trying to act as normal as possible. I just struggled with it. I wore my foot drop braces under my pants, and only got a few questions about them since they were well hidden. I did get more questions about the scar on my neck. Usually these questions came from the kids, but some grown-ups would ask as well. I tried not to let the questions get to me. I knew that unless I was going to wear turtlenecks everyday, I was going to be asked about my scars. When this came up, I would just tell them that my skin there had been sick and needed to be cut out. Then I would tell them they used skin from my legs to cover up the hole. That usually got an "oooooooo" response. I've dealt with that question since and continue to just take it in stride. Some of the kids will even touch one of my grafts, that gets them going even more. Kids speak their minds and are very curious so it's not surprising or inappropriate that they ask.

In October, I began doing some full workdays and later that month I took my first overnight call. When I wasn't working, I was usually resting. Working tired me out so much, I would hit the couch after dinner and was usually snoring before long. Given all that I had been through, it was quite an accomplishment to be working full-time at this point, but I wasn't good for much else. As hard as it was, I was very glad to be contributing at work after my late start.

In terms of my rehab, I saw a physiatrist and an occupational therapist shortly after my arrival in State College. After undergoing some extensive testing, I was basically discharged to do some "home" exercises. The therapist didn't think I needed to come in to the gym to do my rehab. I was disappointed in their analysis, I knew I would get better faster with regular routine therapy like I was doing in Cleveland. With my hours increasing at work, our new baby and our new house we were trying to get established, I knew I wouldn't be good at finding time to exercise regularly at home. I was right. I basically stopped my therapy at that point, only working my shoulder through my activities of daily living.

By the grace of God and not by my own doing, my foot-drop improved after the first few months in Pennsylvania. I would regularly lie on the couch with my feet up over its arm and mentally try to get those toes to move up. One night as I was doing that, my foot suddenly listened, moving the toes up ever so slightly. I was so surprised, I can remember calling Michelle out to see if I was dreaming. She saw it too, this was real. It was only happening in the right foot but we were ecstatic to see some improvement in this area. The right side made steady progress day by day but on the left there was still nothing. The right progressed so much that I finally was able to give up the brace on that foot. Still no progress on the left. We kept praying and I kept trying to will those toes to work when suddenly, they did. Euphoria can't even come close to describing the feelings we had that November night when the left foot started working again. It had taken over six months from the start of my illness for the left side to start working again. It progressed to the point that I gave up my left brace by Christmas. I would still occasionally catch my toes on something if I didn't get my leg up high enough, but the foot-drop totally resolved. I still have some residual numbness on my shins, but otherwise, this went away as everyone had hoped it would. We don't truly understand why this happened and took the time course that it did, but I couldn't have been more thankful to recover from the foot-drop, another step in the long line of miracles.

Though the final surgery had been deemed a success, this didn't mean that trouble with my grafts was over. Shortly after moving to Pennsylvania, I had a small spot open up in my left armpit. This was located right next to the full thickness graft from my forearm where it met another skin graft. It couldn't have been in a more difficult place either. None of us really knew why, I wasn't sure if I had actually torn it open using my left arm or if it just appeared. I talked to Dr. Frat on the phone about it and we started dressing it again. Instead of the two sides healing together, my body started filling the gap with something called granulation tissue. This tissue is very delicate, easily bleeding and not helpful for healing the two sides together. Michelle was forced to start using some chemical cautery sticks with Silver Nitrate to knock that tissue back in hopes of promoting the two sides to come together. Michelle was really concerned about this getting infected so she was working on it every day. I refused to have bandages all around my neck so we resorted to taping the bandage directly on my grafts. If I didn't have a bandage over the opening, it would ooze this yellow fluid onto my shirt so going without wasn't an option. We worked with this area for several months until winter time came and it finally healed. It seemed hot and sweaty areas like armpits are not conducive to the healing process. How nice it was once it healed for good, or so we thought. The same spot opened up slightly the next summer but we were able to heal that quicker and now there appears to be enough scar tissue to keep it together permanently. I have also had several little red and swollen spots along the edges of my grafts flare up. This happened as recently as the summer of 2004. These spots usually end up being small pieces of suture that were left behind. Michelle will open them up, letting out pus and the small piece of suture. This has happened five or six times over the four years. It seems amazing to me that it is still occurring. I also have a couple staples that can be seen underneath the graft, but so far these have not given me any trouble. Despite these little setbacks, I have been so fortunate to have "good" grafts. The doctors always comment on how nice they have turned out, they don't get dried out and cracked like some people's do. I have no idea what the grafts will look like in fifty years, but I hope to be around to see. They aren't pretty now so I guess it doesn't matter much, just as long as they do their job and keep me from spilling out all over.

The doctors have talked to me about doing some plastic surgery to improve the looks of things. They have ever-improving technology to expand out here, nip and tuck there, to lessen the extent of my deformity. As much as I would like for them to tighten up my belly, I just don't feel right considering it. I was blessed enough to survive the unsurvivable and to come out very functional and happy, how could I dare go under the knife again just to make me look a little better. It wouldn't change the overall appearance, they can't make me look good enough to take my shirt off at the pool. It would just reconstruct a few areas that didn't heal as nicely as they could have. I know it is impossible to tell what my feelings will be in the future but for the most part I am content to stick with what is working now. I have had my fill of bandages, sutures, staples, etc. and don't have any desire to go through any more. My scars are a part of me, a very important part that saved my life and yet have no real significance in who I truly am as a person. I totally understand why some people would undergo surgery to improve their looks, things might be different if my scars were in different places. It is an individual decision and one that I am comfortable with. I know that my family and friends would support me if I changed my mind, but they wouldn't love me any more or less if I did, so plastic surgery doesn't make sense to me. If you know someone who is disfigured and is considering surgery, being understanding and supportive is the way to help them through that, whatever their decision. Everyone's situation is different, there is no right or wrong in these types of circumstances.

As we had progressed through my illness, I continually voiced my goal of golfing again. Early on, it seemed like a long shot. Not losing my arm completely was a miracle in and of itself. Despite the major setback, I was bound and determined to get my shoulder in shape enough to play. I remember once sitting in clinic talking to Frat about golfing when he started to tell me a story about a one-armed golfer he had seen play. He had also seen a blind golfer that was just incredible to watch. I remember being somewhat irritated hearing these stories, I was going to play again. Maybe not well, but I was not interested in being some circus attraction. About nine months after my discharge from the hospital, I finally felt up to try golfing during a trip south to visit my parents and some of our medical school friends. Twice on the trip in March 2001, I actually went out and played, once with my brother Eric and once with my friends Gerry and John. In all honesty, I played terribly, but the pure joy of getting out on the golf course was impossible to convey. After such a long battle with the "flesh-eating" bacteria and its residual effects, I had obtained one of my recovery goals. Getting well enough to get back out on the golf course was one of the things I had long been hoping for throughout my illness. The range of motion in my shoulder was significantly hampered, but I was able to put the ball in play, and out of play. With both of these rounds, I didn't care as much as I usually did about being badly beaten. I was competing against myself and was winning just by being out there. After playing, my shoulder joint was extremely sore from working it to the max, but the pain was well worth the sheer accomplishment.

Along with the goal of being able to golf again, another goal was to golf with Dr. Frat. We had discussed it frequently as I laid in my hospital bed, and I finally got the chance to play with him on a return trip to Cleveland during the summer of 2001. He invited me to play at Acacia Country Club, his club of many years. Even though I had been steadily improving since my initial debut in March, I played terribly that day. I was disappointed in my poor effort but thrilled to show the good doctor what an amazing job he had done, giving my shoulder the needed mobility to play. I vowed that we would get a rematch and we were fortunate enough to do that in the summer of 2003. As if totally opposite of the first time I played with him, I played my best round by far since I had been sick. I felt bad for Dr. Frat that day, he didn't have his best game and I actually beat him. It was sure nice of him to let his crippled patient win. Over the years, my swing has improved as my shoulder range of motion has increased, now almost to a full swing. I don't hit the ball as far as I used to, but the ten or twenty yards really doesn't make much difference. Every year my shoulder gets stronger and I feel more comfortable on the golf course. An interesting result of my reconstructed shoulder is that I usually play better on the back nine. It seems to take a long time for my shoulder to get completely loosened up.

Our family has grown again since my illness. On November 11th 2002, Lydia Grace Collison was born at Centre Community Hospital, now known as the Mount Nittany Medical Center. I had been somewhat worried about my ability to father another child after all the stress, medications and radiation that I had been through. Did all these things put us at risk to be infertile, or worse, to have a child with significant birth defects? Despite my reservations, we had always planned on having four children so after talking and praying about it, we

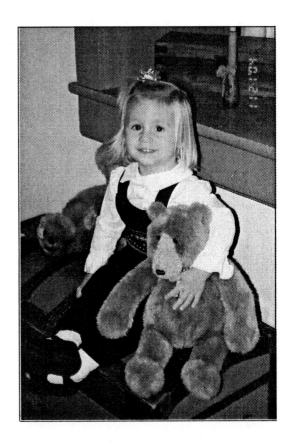

Lydia Grace Collison, age 2.

decided to go ahead. Everything went as if nothing had ever happened. Michelle got pregnant as soon as we started trying, and Lydia was born as "normal" as a Collison can be. Michelle's pregnancy had been difficult, but nothing we couldn't handle. We had the perfect family now, two boys and two girls. It is hard to imagine that Lydia would never have been born had I not survived my terrible illness. I am very thankful that I have this book to share with her as she gets older, to give her a better understanding of why her dad looks the way he does and why her very life and existence are special gifts to us from God.

Being a Pediatrician has its ups and downs as well. It would be hard to come up with a more rewarding job, and I love what I do the majority of time. It can be incredibly stressful too. Some days I struggle with it, taking every parent's burdens onto yourself can be draining. I have been fortunate to work with some exceptional doctors, nurses and support staff. I can't tell you how many times I was told by the nurses and doctors who worked on me while I was sick how beneficial my illness would be for me as a physician. I hope that it has made me a better doctor and person, I'm always trying to pull positives from the difficult experience I went through. I certainly have been in my patient's shoes and can empathize better than most physicians can. My hope is that all my patients feel as though I give them my best.

Now our life is pretty well a normal one. Michelle is homeschooling the boys and keeping extremely busy trying to teach, watch the girls, keep the laundry going and keep us fed. We have become active at church and participate in seemingly countless activities as the kids get older. I am fortunate to be physically able to help coach the boy's little league baseball teams and play football with them in the backyard. Were it not for putting this book together, I might go days without thinking about my illness at all. The effects of it are still there though, every time I look in the mirror, I see the many scars from that dreadful summer of 2000. The chance to put this book together has been such a blessing for me. It has given me the chance to work through all the emotions that come from such an experience. My personality is one that works best if I have goals in front of me to strive toward. I have been persistent at working at it over lunch-breaks and on rainy days for a couple of years now. That longing for a purpose, a reason to justify my illness has also been very healthy for me. It sure beats focusing on the negative results. I've tried, that doesn't help at all. I also have a record of the events now, so that the summer of 2000 will always be remembered, even as the most vivid memories fade with time. By sharing our story, my hope all along has been to help and encourage others in similar circumstances; for the reader to benefit from my pain; to make good on God's investment in keeping me around. I'll keep working toward that. I will hope for your good health, strong faith and a resilient spirit to face the trials of your life.

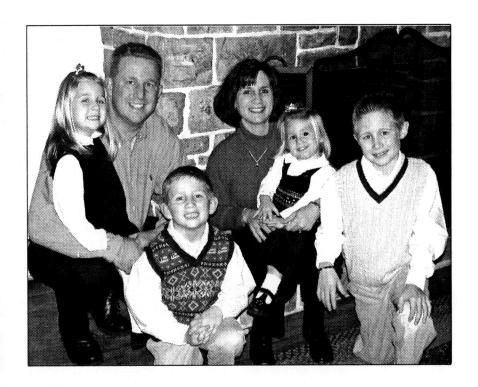

The Collison Family, December 2004.

𝕽omans 6:23 "𝕱or the wages of sin is death, but the gift of 𝕲od is eternal life in 𝕮hrist 𝕵esus our 𝕷ord."

Special Thanks

I am forever indebted to Dr. Goldstein and all the doctors and nurses at University Hospitals of Cleveland for saving my life with their incredible care.

Thank you to Dr. Nieder and all the residents, doctors, nurses and support staff from Rainbow who helped us in so many ways. This goes especially to John and Leron, your support for Michelle will never be forgotten.

I want to thank Dr. Fratianne for writing such a thoughtful foreword, and for our friendship. It means so much to me. The care from Dr. Fratianne, Dr. Yowler, Dr. Kaufman and Dr. Lacey was world-class, as are all the nurses and therapists of the Metrohealth Burn Unit. Thanks to all of you for your efforts in my recovery.

Thank you to everyone I've mentioned in the book who came and visited us in Cleveland. Thanks to all who sent cards and gifts, we appreciated them all. I especially want to thank everyone who prayed for us, even those we've never met. Your prayers were answered.

Thanks to everyone at CMSA who stuck with me and gave the time I needed to recover.

I want to thank my parents, coaches and teachers for molding me into the person that I have become. I can look back now and see how fortunate I have been to be mentored by so many great people. I hope I have made you proud.

Thank you to all of you who are a big part of my life now. The people I work with, "play" with, go to church with, I feel very blessed to be surrounded with so many great people.

I also want to thank my "team" for their help in shaping my ideas and making this book a reality.
Lead Editor: Kimberly Bair
Content Editors: Michelle, Clarence and Sally Collison, Carolyn Foust, Gerry and Christy Dey, Dan Smith
Photography: Michelle, Jamie McCloskey
Cover: Doug Irwin

Thanks Taylor, Chase, Caroline and Lydia for sharing the computer and letting Daddy get this done.

Thank you Michelle, for believing in me and this book, and most of all for your love... C

I would welcome your thoughts on this book. Please send comments to:

Craig H. Collison, MD
Stone House Press
PO Box 36
Madisonburg, PA 16852

Or email comments to: stonehousepress@msn.com

www.stonehousepress.com

Glossary

Types of physicians:

Allergy-   deal with the science of allergies.

Anesthesia-   these physicians work with patients usually during surgery. They take care of the patient's needs while the surgeon is doing the surgical procedure. They often also work in a critical care setting.

Critical Care-   these physicians work in intensive care units managing complex medical issues.

Cardiology-   these physicians work specifically with the heart.

Dermatology-   these physicians deal with issues of the skin.

Endocrinology-   these physicians work with all the hormones in our body, such as the thyroid and adrenal hormones. They also work with with diabetes, obesity, and pubertal problems.

**Family Practice/
General Practitioner-** these physicians take care of primary care issues for patients of all ages.

Gastroenterology- these physician's work with issues of the stomach, liver, gallbladder, pancreas, and bowel.

Geriatrics- these physicians are trained in internal medicine with special training to work with the elderly.

Hematology- these doctors work with issues of the blood.

Nephrology- these doctors work with issues of the kidneys.

Neurology- these doctors work with the brain, spinal cord, and peripheral nervous system.

**Obstetrics and
Gynecology-** these doctors work with women to include care of pregnant women, delivering babies, and any diseases of the female reproductive organs.

Oncology- these doctors work with cancers of all types.

Pathology- these doctors are specifically trained to study body tissues, and perform autopsies.

Pediatrics-	these doctors provide primary medical care for children from birth through adolescence.
Physical Medicine (Physiatry)-	these doctors work with rehabilitation, and other physical disabilities.
Pulmonary-	these doctors work with the lungs and breathing.
Pharmacology-	these doctors work specifically with medications and their effects on patients.
Rheumatology-	these doctors work with autoimmune and joint diseases such as lupus and rheumatoid arthritis.

Surgery

General

Orthopedics-	bones, muscle, ligaments and tendons
Otolaryngology(ENT)-	ear, nose, and throat, also neck
Pediatric-	children
Urology-	genitals and urinary tract
Neurosurgery-	brain, spinal cord and peripheral nerves
Cardiothoracic-	heart and lungs

Trauma

Medical Terms

Chemotherapy- these are medicines specifically aimed at cancer cells and also some autoimmune disorders.

Radiation Therapy- this is therapy to kill cancer cells directly with beams of radiation.

EKG (ECG)- also known as an electrocardiogram, this measures the electrical activity of the heart. This can be interpreted to find arrhythmias, and has characteristic changes in heart attacks and increased heart size.

Echocardiogram- this is test which uses sound waves to image the heart. This can be done in real-time means that it can watch the motion of the heart, and the motion of the blood traveling through the heart. This is done by a probe placed on the outside of the chest wall, or can be done through the esophagus, which is known as a TEE (Trans-Esophageal Echocardiogram).

Swan-Ganz Catheter- this is a catheter which is placed through an artery or vein in your shoulder and then advanced into the heart. This gives very detailed information about pressures and volumes of the blood traveling through the heart, and is very helpful in times of critical illness.

Pulsox- this is a non-invasive way to measure of the oxygen saturation of the blood. The probe is usually placed on the finger or toe, and it uses light sensors to get a reading of the oxygen saturation of the blood.

Intubation- this is the process for placing a breathing tube and through the vocal cords into the trachea. Once the breathing tube is in place this is usually hooked up to a ventilator.

Chest Tube- this tube is placed in-between the ribs into the actual chest cavity. This is done when the lung has collapsed and also when there is blood or other fluid compressing the lungs.

Foley Catheter- this catheter is placed into the bladder which allows the bladder to drain without patients having to urinate.

IV- this is a small catheter which is placed into a vein to provide access to give fluids and/or medicines. This is placed there with a needle which after placement is removed out of the catheter.

Central Line- this is similar to the IV except that it is placed in larger vessels and then threaded close to the heart (central circulation).

CBC-   this stands for complete blood count and looks at white blood cells, red blood cells, platelets, and other values associated with these. A differential can be done with the CBC, and this part of the test gives the percentages of the different types of white blood cells present.

Bone Scan-   this test is a nuclear test which is done by putting special bone-specific contrast into the body through an IV. The scanner then picks up areas in bone that have increased activity or turnover as more contrast travels to these areas.

Cardiac Catheterization- this involves putting a special device through the groin up into the heart. There it measures pressures and volumes and is able to squirt dye into the heart so the anatomy can be well delineated by x-rays as the blood flows through.

Monitor-   is something that is connected to the patient by leads and gives information on heart rate respiratory rate and pulsox. It also can give information on continuous blood pressure readings if an arterial line has been placed.

EEG –   this test involves measuring the electrical activity of the brain. Many electrodes are placed all around the scalp which then record the electrical activity for analysis. This test is often used when there is concern for seizures or lack of brain activity.

CT Scan- this scan is taken by moving in your body through a narrow tube which emits x-rays from all directions. Computer results of these give a cross-section of the person's body part that is being evaluated. Because of the multiple x-rays used, the images that it produces are superior to a standard x-ray.

MRI Scan- this scan is taken by putting your body into a long tube and passing magnetic fields through it. This scan is the most sensitive and accurate for soft tissue evaluation. It often takes 30 to 45 minutes for this scan. It is a difficult scan for people who are claustrophobic. Now there are "open" MRI's available to help with this problem. The other complaint with the MRI scan is a loud, banging noise which is heard by the person in the tube.

Endoscopy- this test involves putting a very small camera on the end of a small tube which is found passed down the esophagus and into the stomach. The tool may also take small biopsies. The patient is sedated during this procedure.

Sedation- this is done by chemical means to put the patient in a semi-conscious state. This is different than anesthesia were the patient is completely asleep.

Anesthesia- this is normally done by inhalation of special gases which render the patient unconscious, usually for surgical or otherwise invasive procedures.

DVT- this stands for deep venous thrombosis. These are clots which form typically in the deep veins of the legs. These can break off and then travel through the heart and block off a blood supply to a section of lung. When this happens, the clot is known as a pulmonary embolism.

Stroke- a stroke occurs when a clot moves up into the brain and blocks its blood supply. This can cause defects in speech and movement, and is typically one-sided as only one side of the brain is affected. If the stroke occurs in the brainstem it is usually deadly as these are the respiratory centers and necessary to coordinate breathing.

Cancer- this general term refers to any disease where the patient's own body tissue loses its control mechanisms and grows out of control, usually creating a tumor. This can be treated by surgery, chemotherapy and radiation therapy.

Skin Graft-   this is where the top layer of skin is taken from healthy skin, and placed to cover defects caused by burns or other trauma.

Defibrillator-   this machine supplies an electric charge to the heart, attempting to change an abnormal rhythm to a regular one.

Abscess-   this is a collection of pus that can be found in almost any part of the body.

Appendix

Intensive Care Units: In larger hospitals, multiple types the intensive care unit's are seen. In contrast, most community hospitals only have one general intensive care unit which attempts to covers as many of these specialties as possible. Below is a list of the most common types of intensive care unit's and their abbreviations.

BICU-   Burn ICU

CICU-   Cardiac ICU

SICU-   Surgical ICU, in very large hospitals this can be further split into specialties such as trauma, neurosurgery, etc.

MICU-   Medical ICU

PICU-   Pediatric ICU

NICU-   Neonatal ICU

For those of you who have never been in an ICU, it is a place where medical technology meets the most serious illness, keeping people alive with technology when they would otherwise be unable to survive. This is the locale where the newest and most

157

experimental therapies are tried and used in a last effort to thwart death. The ICU is also the scariest place for patients and for families as the critical nature of the treatments and the not so infrequent failure to keep patients alive makes it an extremely stressful environment.

An ICU is most frequently designed as a large open area with several beds scattered around a central nursing workstation. Being inside the ICU always reminded me of being in a spacecraft, totally surrounded by machines and computers. Privacy in the ICU is definitely at a minimum, with your only barriers being flimsy curtains or glass walls and sliding glass doors. The lighting is often dim but that is the only thing peaceful about it. Everywhere you look there are machines and monitors with flashing lights and beeping alarms. Most of the time there is at least one patient on a ventilator, so it is easy to hear the constant whish-whoosh of the breathing that is forced in and out of the patient's lungs. For the small area of size the ICU is, there are many more staff packed in as each nurse typically has one to three patients in contrast to regular hospital floors where the ratio is much larger. I was one of those critically ill patients, with one nurse devoted entirely to my care. All of these characteristics make it an intimidating place, and patients and their families are often overwhelmed with the complexity, the many rules, the restricted visitation, and most vividly the critical nature of their loved one's illness. It can be very disheartening to know that everything is being done for your loved one at this level of care, and failure for that care to work results in their death.

The staff of the ICU is composed of many physicians, therapists, nurses, social workers, unit secretaries, clergy, and a very busy cleaning staff. Most ICU's have an "intensivist" who is ultimately in charge of every patient in the ICU. They may come from several different backgrounds, including anesthesia, pulmonary, critical care, and surgery. For more specialized ICU's, there are specially trained physicians who run them as well. An example of this would be a neonatologist being in charge of the neonatal intensive care unit (NICU). The ICU team leader is rarely the only physician involved in each patient's care, normally being surrounded by fellows and residents in a teaching hospital, and also by other specialists depending on the patient's particular ailment.

The therapists who work on the team are specially trained to help with patients in such critical states, and have a much different role than therapists do in an outpatient setting. They often spend time working on things like passive range of motion to keep the patient's joints from getting stiff. Most ICU patients aren't in a condition to work on walking or other gross motor activities due to their degree of illness.

The nurses who work in an ICU are specially trained to work with all the high-tech equipment and often have to coordinate multiple medical therapies at one time. They are constantly at the bedside, providing constant monitoring looking for any changes in their patient's condition.

The ICU social workers are extremely crucial in helping patients and their families as they deal with all of their non-medical issues. This can include housing for the patient's family, help with financial, insurance and logistical issues, finding community based resources depending on the specific family needs, and also placement of the patient once they leave the ICU.

Child-life therapists play a big role in helping children in pediatric ICU's, and also help the children of adults who are patients in any ICU. The child-life therapists from Rainbow did a great job helping everyone know how to talk with Taylor and Chase during the beginning of my illness. They also provided gifts for the children, and gave me a quilt that had been donated in an attempt to brighten my room in the ICU.

The unit secretaries are the managers of the ICU logistics. In my experience they see all, know all, and are crucial to an efficient and successful ICU. They manage all the phone calls coming in and out, they order tests, often on an emergent basis, and manage the in and outflows of everyone from families to physicians in the ICU. Most of the time visitors need to buzz in and obtain permission from the unit secretary to gain admission, depending on if the patient can be seen or not.

Clergy are very active in the ICU as well, and are very good at helping support the families regardless of religious backgrounds. They have to be comfortable with death to work in such a stressful environment. In talking with my pastor now, he related to me a strategy used to train clergy for medical or difficult situations in general. It is known as a "ministry of presence." The theory is that just being there is helpful and supportive for those in need. Are there really words that can help the situation as a human being is dying? The support of having someone there to lean on and cry on is often more valuable than words.

Last but not least, all good ICU's have a very active cleaning crew. Since ICU's are where the sickest patients are cared for, the bacteria that are found in them tend to be the most aggressive and resistant. Since bacteria get everywhere, patients already seriously ill are highly susceptible to "iatrogenic" infections from these nasty bacteria. Iatrogenic in basic terms means the infection was caused by being in the hospital rather than from being caught by chance out in the community. Aggressive cleaning and disinfecting are crucial to keeping patients as safe as possible. ICU cleaning crews do an incredible job at this.

Pain Medications:

My suggestion in regards to the use of pain medications is to use them as long as you need to, and not a minute more. Anyone taking narcotics must beware of becoming too dependent on them. Some people are more at risk for this than others, and you never know how your body will respond to pain medicines until you try them. I disliked the way they made me feel so it was never a concern to me, but I have seen so many people suffer from addiction and dependence on these medications. Getting off of pain medications at the appropriate time gives one such a great feeling, both from your clearer head and the accomplishment of an improving condition.

Tylenol (acetominophen): this is a common pain reliever which works both for pain and for reducing fever. Tylenol is easy on the stomach and metabolized by the liver. As well tolerated as Tylenol is, it can be deadly in overdose situations.

Non-Steroidal Anti-Inflammatory Drugs (NSAIDS): these are also common pain relievers which work both for pain and reducing fever. These medicines are more difficult on the stomach than Tylenol but normally well-tolerated. These drugs, most commonly ibuprofen and naprosyn, are metabolized by the kidneys. They can cause trouble in dehydrated patients due to decreased blood flow to the kidney in the dehydrated state.

Narcotics: these drugs work in the brain to to block specific pain receptors. These drugs can be addicting and must be controlled carefully. These drugs also have significant side effects including constipation and respiratory depression. Examples of these medicines include Morphine, Demerol, Vicodin and Percocet.

Anxiolytics: these drugs also work in the brain and act basically to calm and also to erase the memory of anything that happens while the patient is under the influence of this drug. These drugs also have side effects including respiratory depression. Examples of these medicines include Valium, Xanax and Ativan.

Breathing: this technique was made most popular by the Lamaze and Bradley methods of breathing during childbirth. The breathing is a way to move the focus away from the pain and onto the effort of breathing.

Distraction: this technique is used very frequently with children and is another way to take the "mind" off of the pain. There are specialists who work in a field known as child life who are experts at reading to children, playing games, and doing entertaining things while children are undergoing painful procedures. Similar techniques can also work with adults.

Emergency Room

Most people can relate to a trip to the Emergency Room at some point in their lives, usually under difficult circumstances. There are also several television shows that have shown a glamorized or real-life Emergency Room. The Emergency Room serves several purposes in our health-care system. Most importantly it provides emergency care of trauma and sudden onset-illnesses. It is also a conduit into the hospital itself. The ER is a place where patients being admitted are assessed and stabilized prior to going to their hospital room. The third function of Emergency Rooms in our society is that of primary care to people who don't have a physician and/or insurance. This is an expensive and inefficient way to take care of a patient's non-emergent care, but it continues to occur on a daily basis in almost every Emergency Room across the country.

Everyone's experience in an Emergency Room begins with registration. Personal information is obtained, including any existing insurance information. Once they are registered in the hospital system, each patient is assessed and triaged unless they come by ambulance. In most cases, those patients coming by ambulance usually take first priority. Triage is the process of medically-trained personnel determining each patient's degree of illness and subsequently giving them a priority status. This way the doctors know who the sickest patients are and can attend to them first.

In the general Emergency Room scenario, once a patient has been entered into the system and placed in a room or bed, the doctor or provider does the initial assessment. This includes questions regarding the patient's condition and a physical exam. Using the results of this information, the physician establishes a differential diagnosis, in basic terms a list of potential causes for the patient's condition. This list can be very simple, as in the case of a laceration (cut), or very complex when multiple injuries have occurred or only non-specific symptoms are seen. From this list of potential causes, a plan of action to determine the diagnosis and any-needed supportive measures are undertaken. In today's high-tech world of medicine, the number of potential tests available to an emergency room physician is staggering.

The next phase of an Emergency Room visit is usually a waiting game, waiting for labs and x-rays and other tests to be run and the results to be analyzed. This wait can be very agonizing, but seems to be a necessary part of any trip to the emergency room. Once the results from the various tests are available, then the decisions are made regarding treatment. It is also decided at this time whether or not the patient needs to be admitted or transferred to another medical facility, such as a nursing home or large referral center.

The keys to having a successful visit to the Emergency Room are these:

1. Be your own advocate - You must stand up for yourself or your loved one and get them the attention they need. The ER is a busy place, let those taking care of you know what is needed in a kind and respectful way.

2. Ask questions - Keep asking questions until you understand the situation on your level so you can make informed decisions.

3. Be patient - tests take a while to run and the staff of the ER are always stretched between many patients so keeping your patience will keep everyone's stress level to a minimum.

While the Emergency Room is a challenging, confusing and often frustrating place to receive medical care, as a whole, the emergency medicine system in our country does a good job treating sudden illness and trauma. It also works well as an access route to further medical care including inpatient admission. It can also provide non-emergent care, though primary care physicians in an office setting do a much better job with these issues. Our society owes a great debt to the physicians and staff working in our emergency departments, saving lives with critical decision-making under incredible stress. This happens 24 hours a day, 365 days a year across the country, and we as a society can only hope that this coverage will continue indefinitely.

Hospital Day

There is a patterned schedule that most people experience when they are in the hospital. This pattern of activity is followed not for the convenience of the patients and families but rather to facilitate physicians seeing their patients early in the day, so that they can get to their other responsibilities. This is different from an ICU as the doctors aren't necessarily on the unit. The treatments and therapies that the physicians order during their early morning rounds can then be carried out by ancillary staff during daylight hours. This isn't always the most convenient timing for anyone but the physicians, but this is just the way things typically work in the hospital.

In discussing perhaps the most important schedule in terms of patient care, I will start with the nurses. They typically work either eight or 12 hour shifts. The eight hours shifts I've seen most often go from 7 AM to 3 PM, 3 PM to 11 PM, and 11 PM to 7 AM. When 12 hour shifts are used, the typically go from 7 AM to 7 PM, then 7 PM to 7 AM. Changes in nursing staff are a big deal to patients and their families, as they spend so much of their day dealing directly with their nurse. Having a new nurse every eight hours can be very frustrating, but is unfortunately part of the medical system we have. Having the same nurse for 12 hours can sometimes be very helpful as you get to know someone better, and you have less change in routines.

Then sometime in the early morning, the physicians and medical team will round on all their patients. Rounding is the term used to describe the process where physicians and staff go room to room, examining each patient and looking at laboratory studies and any other information that is available. Once all the information is gathered, the team makes decisions regarding the patient's care for that day. By the time that the rounds are over, the patient and family should have a good idea what will be going on during the day. Sometime during this rounding process, breakfast will come, which can be difficult to eat since the patient is often interrupted much of this early morning time. As difficult as it is for some families to be present during this time, it is definitely the most informative chance to figure out what is happening with the patient's progress and plans. At other points during the day, it is always more difficult to speak with one of the physicians, especially if they are at the office or in the operating room. I strongly suggest that every effort be made for those interested to be present with the patient at this time of day. In more intensive care situations, the physicians are actually in the unit the majority of the day, and being present for morning rounds is not as crucial.

Rehabilitation

The folks who work in the various fields of rehabilitation usually have the word therapist at the end of their title, examples being physical therapists, occupational therapists, speech therapists, etc. Nutritionists also play a role in rehabilitation, as they do during all illnesses. The differences between physical and occupational therapists are sometimes difficult to distinguish, but in basic terms occupational therapists work with fine motor skills (small movements) and activities of daily living while physical therapists work more with gross motor activities and ambulation (walking with or without assistance). They usually work together to help rebuild and re-teach what the illness or injury has taken away from the patient.

There is a large deal of skill involved in being a great therapist. It is not easy for any therapist to push a patient enough to make progress, without going too far. The goal is to help the patient deal with the pain without the patient losing respect for the therapist. As humans, we all have a breaking point past which we can no longer progress, but rather we close up and give up. Finding a balance between pushing enough for improvement while keeping the patient with a positive attitude requires continual evaluation and adjustment from the therapist.

---

[1] Stevens Dennis L, The Flesh Eating Bacterium What's Next The Journal of Infectious Diseases. 1999: 179(Suppl. 2):S366-74.

Printed in the United States
27214LVS00001B/16-75

9 781595 261694